UEHIRO SERIES IN PRACTICAL ETHICS

General Editor: Julian Savulescu, University of Oxford

———

BEYOND HUMANITY?

D0924489

UEHIRO SERIES IN PRACTICAL ETHICS

General Editor: Julian Savulescu, University of Oxford

BEYOND HUMANITY?

THE ETHICS OF BIOMEDICAL ENHANCEMENT

ALLEN BUCHANAN

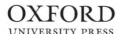

OXFORD
UNIVERSITY PRESS

OXFORD

UNIVERSITY PRESS

Great Clarendon Street, Oxford, OX2 6DP,
United Kingdom

Oxford University Press is a department of the University of Oxford.
It furthers the University's objective of excellence in research, scholarship,
and education by publishing worldwide. Oxford is a registered trade mark of
Oxford University Press in the UK and in certain other countries

© Allen Buchanan 2011

The moral rights of the author have been asserted

First published 2011
First published in paperback 2013

Impression: 1

British Library Cataloguing in Publication Data

Data available

Library of Congress Cataloging in Publication Data

Data available

ISBN 978-0-19-958781-0 (hbk.)
978-0-19-967149-6 (pbk.)

Printed in Great Britain by
MPG Books Group, Bodmin and King's Lynn

THE UEHIRO SERIES IN PRACTICAL ETHICS

In 2002 the Uehiro Foundation on Ethics and Education, chaired by Mr Eiji Uehiro, established the Uehiro Chair in Practical Ethics at the University of Oxford. The following year the Oxford Uehiro Centre for Practical Ethics was created within the Philosophy Faculty. Generous support by the Uehiro Foundation enabled the establishment of an annual lecture series, The Uehiro Lectures in Practical Ethics. These three lectures, given each year in Oxford, capture the ethos of the Oxford Uehiro Centre for Practical Ethics: to bring the best scholarship in analytic philosophy to bear on the most significant problems of our time. The aim is to make progress in the analysis and resolution of these issues to the highest academic standard in a manner that is accessible to the general public. Philosophy should not only create knowledge, it should make people's lives better. Books based upon the lectures are published by Oxford University Press in the Uehiro Series in Practical Ethics.

Julian Savulescu
Uehiro Chair in Practical Ethics
Director, Oxford Uehiro Centre for Practical Ethics, University of Oxford
Editor, The Uehiro Series in Practical Ethics

for Sandy

CONTENTS

PREFACE

Human beings have always tried to enhance themselves—to improve their mental, physical, and emotional capacities. The invention of writing, for example, was a dramatic enhancement of our cognitive powers; the development of the method and practices of science was another. But for the first time we have scientific knowledge that has the potential for transforming ourselves perhaps more profoundly—and certainly more deliberately—than ever before.

Biomedical enhancements achieve improvements in our capacities by working directly on the brain or body. There are several modes of biomedical enhancement: the administration of drugs, implants using genetically engineered tissue, direct brain–computer interface technologies, and insertion of genes into human embryos. Emerging technologies have the potential to transform our very biology.

Biomedical enhancements are already here and more are on the way. Drugs that were developed to treat Alzheimer's dementia, narcolepsy, and attention deficit disorder have been shown to improve normal thinking. Students, professors, and executives are already taking them for that purpose. Direct brain–computer interface technologies are being developed to help people who have lost their vision or control over their limbs and this research will inevitably lead to possibilities for enhancing normal functions. New prosthetic limbs are already out-performing flesh and blood legs—and being banned from running competitions. Genetic engineering techniques applied to laboratory animals are already quite sophisticated and in principle they could be applied to humans. Because enhancements are an inevitable spin-off of advances in the treatment of disease, the choice of whether to use them or not is unavoidable.

A first reaction to the prospect of biomedical enhancements may be: "Why not? Isn't it better to be better?" But on reflection a thicket of ethical issues quickly comes into view. Could biomedical enhancements—especially those employing genetic engineering—result in our being something other than human? Is it wrong to change human nature? What would it mean to change human nature? Will biomedical technologies help "level the playing field" by giving a boost to those at the low end of the normal distribution of intelligence or emotional well-being, or will they make existing inequalities worse? Will the pursuit of enhancements become an endless quest for perfection and make us unappreciative of what we already have?

These are some of the questions explored in this volume. The approach to them is distinctive in several ways. For one thing, my approach takes evolutionary biology seriously. I argue that much of the opposition to biomedical enhancement rests on a gross misunderstanding of evolution. An understanding of evolution is necessary, both to see how beneficial enhancements could be and to appreciate their real risks and to pursue them in a responsible manner. For another, I go beyond the deadlock of exchanging "pros" and "cons" regarding enhancement and move on to what should be the next stage of the debate: trying to figure out effective, realistic institutional responses to the challenges of enhancement.

CHAPTER ONE

The Landscape of the Enhancement Debate

[handwritten: side of B.E. that is very interesting to me. What would this look like & entail?]

Biotechnologies already on the horizon will enable us to be smarter, have better memories, be stronger, quicker, have more stamina, live longer, be more resistant to diseases, and enjoy richer emotional lives. To some of us, these prospects are heartening; to others, they are dreadful. The following statement is typical of those who greet the prospect of enhancement with trepidation.

For the first time, human biology and even the human genome itself can be shaped by human action. But the human organism is a finely balanced whole, the product of eons of exacting evolution. It is irresponsible to tamper with the wisdom of nature, the handiwork of the Master Engineer of evolution, in order to be better than well. Our situation at present is not perfect, of course, but it is clearly satisfactory; so it is a mistake to risk it for the sake of improvement. Those who seek biomedical enhancement desire perfection; they crave mastery. But such attitudes are incompatible with a due appreciation of the given, a sense of gratitude for what we have.[1]

[handwritten: perfection vs. gratitude? Interesting relationship]

This way of framing the enhancement issue may be initially appealing. Unfortunately, it happens to be dead wrong. More precisely: *each and every sentence in the above passage above is false* and in the remainder of this book I will demonstrate that this is so. Here, a preview of my findings will suffice. Human action has shaped human biology and altered the genome as long as there have been human beings: a series of non-biomedical enhancements of human capacities, from the agrarian revolution, to the emergence of cities and political institutions, to *stated as a fact, feels like an opinion, depends on what harmonious & "complete" means to the individual.*

advances in transportation technologies, has triggered processes of natural selection and mixed previously isolated gene pools. The human organism is not a finely balanced whole, because evolution does not create harmonious, "complete" organisms; instead it produces tentative, changing, perishing, cobbled-together *ad hoc* solutions to transient design problems, with blithe disregard for human well-being. Nature is not wise (or unwise) and evolution is not like a Master Engineer; it is more like a morally insensitive, blind, tightly shackled tinkerer. The situation of millions of human beings is *not* satisfactory, and both to improve their lives and to preserve the well-being of the most fortunate among us it may be necessary to undertake biomedical enhancements. To solve problems we have created—such as environmental pollution, over-population, and global warming—human beings may have to enhance their cognitive capacities and perhaps their moral capacities as well. The pursuit of biomedical enhancements is not the pursuit of perfection; it is the pursuit of improvement. To desire to enhance certain human capacities in order to increase human well-being or to preserve the well-being we now enjoy is not the same as desiring to achieve total mastery. A proper appreciation of the given is compatible with the pursuit of improvement and may require enhancement, if enhancement is needed to preserve what is valuable in the given. → *the given is an*

The debate about biomedical enhancements is one of the most exciting and frustrating controversies of our time. Exciting, because it raises the most enduring questions: about what it is to be human, about individuality, about our relationship to nature, and about what sort of society we should strive to have. Frustrating, because the quality of the debate is low, in five respects.

okay, but true

interesting & successful affect on my view of life & science as "magic." Doesn't sound so magical when it is put that way

did thin abt thi optio

eb flow not preserv

mindset only some will maintain, some will pursue "perfection"

1. *Murky rhetoric masquerading as argument*

First, perhaps more so than in any other area of ethical controversy, some of the most prominent figures in the debate persistently substitute high-sounding rhetoric for reasoning. This is not a peripheral annoyance. As I shall show, it infects the central "arguments" of some of the most prominent critics of enhancement—those who appear to reject enhancement *as such*, rather than merely rejecting *some* enhancements, in some circumstances, when undertaken for certain reasons or as the expression of certain values. To my knowledge, there is no other part of the Practical Ethics literature in which academic writers continue, in the face of articulate, fair, and powerful criticism, to deploy grand-sounding, but deeply ambiguous catchphrases and slogans at the heart of their views, and never take the trouble to try to translate them into sound arguments. For example, some writers claim that the pursuit of enhancement betrays a character that is deficient in the virtue of "grati-tude" for "the given,"[2] without even considering that, properly speaking, gratitude is appropriate only in response to a benefit conferred by an agent, and, in particular, a benefit that is intentionally conferred. *gratitude* Nonetheless, these writers claim that the "argument from gratitude" *grateful=* does not rely on the assumption that "the given" is a gift from God.[3] *appreciating* They claim that considerations of "gratitude" provide a powerful objec- *something* tion to enhancement even if the debate is restricted to a public discourse that is accessible to the nonreligious as well as the religious.[4] One might *wouldn't* well feel *fortunate* that the contingencies of evolution have produced a *be that* world in which there is so much color and beauty, but a person who was *confused* grateful to evolution would be confused.

The most serious problem with the appeal to gratitude, however, is *gratitude=* not its careless inaccuracy. It is the yawning gap between the truism that *"pleased* one should recognize that much of what is good in life is not the result of *& relieved"* our efforts, on the one hand, and any practical guidance as to how to face the challenges of enhancement, on the other.

Even if one ought to be appreciative of the good things one has and aware that many of them are unearned, it doesn't follow from this that one should refrain from ever trying to improve one's life or the life of others. For one thing, "the given" includes some pretty dreadful items: ghastly diseases, the deterioration of mental and physical capacities that is part of the "normal" aging process, and human propensities toward violence and exploitation. Why is it permissible to *not* resign ourselves to "bad givens" like horrible diseases? If the answer is that it is permissible to change those "givens" that are departures from "normal functioning" but not others, then another question immediately arises: why is "nor-mal functioning" morally privileged, or off-limits to improvement? — *the issue* Anyone who knows a bit about evolutionary biology and admits that *of class* our thinking about "the natural" should at the very least be consistent *inequality* with evolutionary science will have serious reservations about the as- *maybe?* sumption that normal functioning is sacrosanct.[5] Normal functioning, from the standpoint of evolutionary biology, is simply functioning that is typical of the organism as it happens to be now, as a result of the highly contingent path its species has traversed so far. It is not optimal functioning, and need not be harmonious functioning, good functioning, or even satisfactory functioning—*from the standpoint of what we rightly value*. The italicized qualifier is crucial: all that evolution can be expected to increase, and then only approximately and fleetingly, is reproductive fitness. Fitness in biology refers to the ability to survive and reproduce, a propensity that is not aimed at or in any way indexed to human good. This distinction is of crucial importance. Survival and reproduction might be achieved in a situation where vast numbers of human beings live miserable lives, hovering just above subsistence, under conditions of gross over-population. To confuse human good with what evolution delivers is to miss the point of the Darwinian revolution in biology and to revert to the very teleological view of nature it overthrew.

Given that appreciation of "the given" cannot mean we should never enhance, we need to know which sorts of enhancements, for whom, in what circumstances, undertaken for what reasons, are compatible with this virtue. We also need to know why we should *assume* that appreciation of the given is so overwhelmingly important that we should forgo all of the benefits that enhancements might bring, in order to avoid any deficiency in that virtue. We should also consider the possibility that the contours of a virtue may be determined in part by consideration of such benefits—in other words, that *proper* appreciation of the given must take into account the benefits that would be lost if we were to remain content with "the given" and forgo improvements.

How, exactly, are we supposed to get from the importance of the virtue of gratitude or a proper appreciation of the given to an "argument" against enhancement? It is remarkable that those who make the idea of gratitude central to their criticism of enhancement do not even attempt to answer this question. Instead, they leave us with the impression that their appeal to gratitude enables us to draw a line that excludes enhancements generally from the realm of the ethical. Profound-sounding rhetoric about the virtue of gratitude, acceptance of "the given," or "openness to the unbidden" is no substitute for reasoning to a conclusion about what we should do.

The tendency to substitute rhetoric for argument is not confined to American anti-enhancement writers. The famous German philosopher

Jürgen Habermas simply asserts that one cannot regard oneself as free if one is the "product" of one's parents' genetic engineering. He solemnly declares that

> ...interventions aiming at enhancement...violate the fundamental equal status of persons as autonomous beings...insofar as they tie down the person concerned to rejected, but irreversible intentions of third parties, barring him from the spontaneous self-perception of being the undivided author of his own life.[6]

This passage contains a numbing *non sequitur*. The fact that the parents' intentions to design the genotype of an embryo cannot be reversed after they have been implemented does not imply that the phenotypic characteristics they wished to create by designing it cannot be avoided or reversed. To think otherwise is to indulge in the crudest sort of genetic determinism. If Habermas's assumption is that designing the genotype of an embryo means determining all the characteristics of the individual who develops from that embryo, then he has overlooked entirely the influence of the environment and other important developmental factors, including the fact that at a certain stage of development humans can shape the environment they find themselves in or, in some cases, choose to place themselves in another environment. On this interpretation, Habermas has conflated designing the genotype of an embryo with designing a person. If, instead, his claim is that any significant genetic designing of a human embryo (even if it does not fully determine a person's characteristics) is incompatible with that person *regarding* herself as free, then this is a highly ambiguous statement. It could mean that such an individual could not, as a matter of psychological fact, *regard* herself as free—that thinking of herself as free, if she knew she had developed from a "designed" embryo, would be beyond her capacity. Or it could mean that she could not *correctly* regard herself as free—that she would not *be* free, if she so developed. On the first interpretation, the claim is an example of outmoded, armchair psychology that too often occurs in anti-enhancement writing: in this case, this amounts to simply asserting a vast empirical generalization about what people are and are not capable of thinking, without a shred of evidence to support it. On the second interpretation, it is a philosophical claim that is obviously false. Whether an individual is free doesn't depend upon how she came to be; it depends upon what she is

What if we accidentally mess with that capacity?

like, whether she has the capacities that make one free. An individual who develops the normal capacities that persons have is a person, regardless of whether the genotype of her embryo was designed or came to be in the old-fashioned way; and if persons are free, then she is free. Given how implausible the philosophical claim is, the psychological claim is pretty demeaning: It amounts to the assertion that people are so rigidly attached to genetic determinism, in spite of its rejection by genomic science and developmental biology, that they are unable to understand that whether one is free depends upon what one is like, not upon how the embryo from which one developed came about. If in fact people are such genetic determinists, then the proper course of action would be to help them shed this false belief, and devoting considerable effort to doing so might be warranted if the benefits of genetic interventions in embryos were great enough. Habermas does not even consider possible benefits, however. Instead, he rests content with the bare assertion that if one develops from a genetically designed embryo, one cannot be (or cannot regard oneself?) as free. When it is not backed up with sound reasoning, profound-sounding rhetoric about freedom is just as unhelpful as profound-sounding rhetoric about gratitude.

Sometimes, the rhetoric refers to human nature or the natural, as when we are told that enhancement endangers human nature or shows a mistaken (and morally deficient) orientation toward the natural world.[7] Surprisingly, such assertions are oblivious to the fact that the concepts of human nature and the natural are deeply contested and, since the Darwinian revolution in biology, deeply problematic.[8] Here we come to a second source of frustration: the enhancement debate doesn't take evolutionary biology seriously.[9]

2. *Ignoring evolutionary biology*

To the extent that one relies on claims about human nature to support a position either in favor of or against enhancement, what one says shouldn't contradict the fundamentals of evolutionary biology. This modest stricture, I shall argue in Chapter Four, is routinely violated by influential anti-enhancement writers.

In the twenty-first century, there is no excuse for any moderately well-educated person to regard the concept of human nature as anything but highly problematic.[10] Above all, one ought to be very skeptical about the very idea that the concept of human nature that can do any significant work in the enhancement debate or any other serious moral controversy.

One reason the coherence and usefulness of the concept of human nature is so problematic is that it has traditionally been understood against the background of a naïve and simplistic dichotomy between Nature and Nurture that has now been wholly discredited by a better understanding of the complex relationships between genes and environment and between genotype and phenotype.[11] Another is that there is a vigorous, sophisticated contemporary debate about which widely shared characteristics are "cultural" and which are "biological," or, more accurately, about the extent to which explanations of these characteristics require reference to cultural, as opposed to biological causes. This debate is not new of course, but for the first time it is scientifically informed, by work in comparative psychology, neuroscience, anthropology, evolutionary psychology, and genomics. If human nature means the biologically given, the ongoing dispute about what is cultural and what is biological makes appeals to human nature problematic. Under these conditions, relying on an unexplicated, undefended conception of human nature to support a contested position on enhancement is like using a house of cards to shore up the shaky foundations of a skyscraper. Just as important, given our growing knowledge of the reciprocal influences between biological and cultural evolution,[12] the claim that our nature is our biology is both misleading and, to the extent that it is true, less important.

Prominent participants in the enhancement debate also ignore something that every serious student of Ethics now knows: that it is highly problematic, to put it mildly, to try to derive substantive moral conclusions from any concept of human nature.[13] To the extent that we can make sense of the concept of human nature, and do so in a way that is at least compatible with what we know about evolution, we may be able to say that our nature provides some *constraints* on what could be a defensible morality or a good life for beings like us. Put more positively, our nature no doubt contributes something important to the *general shape* of morality and of the good life for us. It is quite another matter to think that an appeal to human nature can tell us whether we should undertake this or that enhancement or to avoid enhancements altogether. To do that, a concept of human nature would have to reveal quite a lot about the *content* of morality, but there is no reason to believe it can, and a number of good reasons to believe it cannot.

So far as the enhancement debate revolves around claims about human nature and the natural, it reflects a pre-Darwinian view of nature and our place in it. For example, as I shall argue later, when the most vociferous critics of enhancement, including former President Bush's Council on Bioethics, invoke the idea of evolution, they mangle it: they attribute a goodness, harmony, and stability to "the natural" that Darwin went out of his way to repudiate. Darwin's conception of evolution and of the natural as the product of evolution was much darker, as the following quote from his letter to Joseph Hooker indicates: "What a book a Devil's Chaplain might write on the clumsy, wasteful, blundering low and horridly cruel works of nature!"[14]

In Chapters Five and Six, I argue that both the risks and the benefits of enhancement look quite different, depending upon whether one's view of human beings is informed by an accurate understanding of evolutionary biology. If one grasps even the most basic elements of evolutionary biology, one will be much more skeptical about talk of "the wisdom of nature," and less inclined to think that the risks of "interfering with nature" are so great as to rule out all enhancements. Whether the proper analogy for evolution is that of a Master Engineer or that of a blind, morally insensitive, tightly shackled tinkerer makes a considerable difference as to how one thinks about the risk of unintended consequences in the case of inheritable genetic modifications. I will argue that the tinkerer analogy is more apt, but that no analogy can take us far in answering questions about the ethics of biomedical enhancement. Instead, we need to use the scientific knowledge we have about the specific causal relationships that might be disrupted by our interventions in deciding whether or not to pursue a particular enhancement.

3. *Sweeping empirical claims, without evidence*

A third source of frustration in the enhancement debate is that it is often breathtakingly naïve, from a methodological point of view. The problem is not simply that bare assertions are offered where reasoning from premises to conclusion is needed, but also that there often seems to be no awareness of the need for empirical evidence. For example, as I shall argue later, critics of enhancement such as Michael Sandel and Leon

Kass repeatedly make vast empirical generalizations about the psychology of those who pursue enhancement. They assert that to try to enhance is to strive for total mastery of the conditions of human existence and to aim obsessively for perfection, and that those who want to extend human life lust for immortality.[15] Sandel, for example, views genetic engineering as "the ultimate expression of our resolve to see ourselves astride the world, the masters of our nature." But, he contends, our quest for mastery is flawed because it "threatens to banish our appreciation of life as a gift, and to leave us with nothing to affirm or behold outside our own will."[16] These authors try to discredit enhancement *in toto*, rather than just some enhancements under some circumstances, by attributing unseemly motivations to all who want to enhance. In doing so, they show no awareness either of the *prima facie* implausibility of such claims or of the need for evidence to support them. In addition, these writers tend to make sweeping generalizations about the effects of enhancement on social institutions—for example, that they will lead to an extreme stratification of society, undermine solidarity, and erode the commitment to distributive justice.[17] In this regard, the enhancement literature is one of the last academic strongholds of *a priori* psychology and sociology. One would think that one was in living in the eighteenth century, when serious intellectuals still believed they could formulate interesting and controversial generalizations about human behavior or the workings of human society from the armchair.

[handwritten margin note: — I think these are real things to be concerned about]

Consider, for a moment, the claim that all, or even most people, who desire enhancement are motivated by a yearning for total mastery, or perfection, or immortality.[18] To treat this claim as self-evident, which is precisely what those who assert such claims do, is naïve in the extreme. How could anyone deny that some may seek an enhancement in order to be *better* in some particular way without thereby desiring to achieve total mastery of the conditions of life or to be perfect? And why would we think that people cannot desire to live *longer* without craving immortality? Surely the burden of empirical evidence is on those who deny the commonsense notion that the desire for betterment is different from the desire for perfection and that the desire for a longer life is different from the desire to live forever.[19]

Similarly, some anti-enhancement writers simply assert sweeping empirical generalizations about human relationships. For example, they declare that if enhancement through genetic interventions in human embryos becomes widespread then valuable relationships will be seriously damaged or destroyed. Such writers predict that the parent–child relationship will be undermined or distorted because children will come to be (or be regarded as?) manufactured items.[20] They also proclaim that if reproductive cloning is used in the service of enhancement, then the boundary between generations "will become confounded."[21] It is hard to know what to make of such evocative, but vague, rhetoric, but this much is clear: these are very ambitious predictions about what the effects of certain kinds of enhancements will be. But causal predictions are empirical claims and they require evidence. None is provided. Instead, they are apparently regarded by those who make them as self-evidently true, which they clearly are not.

4. *Fundamental unclarity: what's your bottom line?*

Perhaps the greatest problem with the rhetoric of the harshest critics of enhancement is that it is so murky that it makes it very hard to tell exactly what they are arguing for or against. If critics like Sandel, Kass, and Fukuyama are arguing against those who hold that all enhancements, under all conditions, are a good thing, or that our society should plunge headlong, and uncritically, into the pursuit of enhancements, then they are arguing against the flimsiest of strawmen, because no one holds that view. If they are arguing against the view that some enhancements, under some conditions, are permissible—that is, if they are rejecting enhancement across the board—then they are committed to some extraordinarily implausible claims: that everyone, or almost everyone, who desires some particular enhancement is motivated by the desire for total mastery, perfection, or immortality, or that all enhancement is destructive of valuable human relationships or threatens to destroy what is valuable in human beings.

Sometimes, anti-enhancement writers, after indulging in passionate rhetorical exercises that seem to be blanket condemnations of enhancement as such, retreat rather meekly to much weaker and thoroughly uncontroversial claims. For example, quite late in his scathing indictment of enhancement, *The Case Against Perfection*, Michael Sandel abruptly switches to a much more plausible but also much less exciting position in the following passage.

Nor do I claim that people who bioengineer their children or themselves are necessarily motivated by a desire for mastery, and that this motive is a sin no good result could possibly outweigh. I am suggesting instead that the moral stakes in the enhancement debate are not fully captured by the familiar categories of autonomy and rights, on the one hand, and the calculation of costs and benefits, on the other.[22]

Given its context in *Against Perfection*, this passage is astonishing. It amounts to a retraction of his claim that he has offered an "argument against enhancement" as opposed to some considerations about character that should be taken into account in the complex task of deciding what to do about enhancement. It also places Sandel on the horns of a dilemma: either he should stick to his guns and expunge this passage to make it consistent with the general tenor of his book, namely, that the pursuit of enhancements is so morally tainted by its roots in character deficiencies that we should forgo it altogether; or he should admit that he has not provided an "argument against enhancement," but instead has only made the uncontroversial point that considerations of character should be taken into account in deciding what to do about enhancement, while also admitting that he has done nothing to fill the yawning gap between making this point and providing any practical guidance about when we ought and we when ought not to pursue enhancements.[23]

5. Stuck at the "pros and cons" stage

A fifth frustrating characteristic of the current state of the enhancement debate is that it has stalled: after more than 20 years, there is still a torrent of articles and books advancing the pros and cons of enhancement, as if it made sense to be either "for enhancement" or "against enhancement." I shall argue that being for enhancement or against enhancement makes as little sense as being pro-globalization or anti-globalization or, for that matter, being pro-technology or anti-technology. In all three cases, we are faced with a complex but undeniable fact: something momentous is happening on an increasingly large scale, there is every reason to believe it will continue, it is impossible to make sweeping claims about whether its effects are or will be good or bad overall, and there is no realistic prospect of stopping the development in

[handwritten margin note: not productive bc there are pros & cons to everything]

its tracks. Instead, the task is to try to understand the phenomenon in all
its complexity, to resist the tendency toward sweeping condemnation or
praise, and, above all, to start thinking hard about practical responses
that are ethically sensitive, true to the complexity of the phenomena, and
realistic. For fairly obvious reasons, effective responses to enhancement
(and to globalization and technological innovation) will have both an
individual and an institutional component: as individuals we will need
to put our values in order, but we will also need to devise policies, and in
some cases perhaps new institutions, to help ensure that those values are
realized.

The most acerbic opponents of enhancement too often simply point
out what they take to be the dangers of enhancement, leaving the reader
with the impression that the solution is for us to strengthen our moral
fiber, pull up our moral socks, and just say "no." Those who take a more
positive stance toward enhancement acknowledge that there are serious
risks, but they typically say too little about how we should mitigate
them. For example, Jonathan Glover, one of the founders of modern
Practical Ethics and one of the most astute writers on enhancement, says
that we should make sure that our efforts to enhance our children do not
express or worsen "ugly attitudes" toward those with disabilities.[24] His
advice is sound, but doesn't say how we are to achieve the needed moral
restraint.

The emergence of enhancement technologies is an institutional phenomenon: so far biomedical enhancements have appeared within a
framework of research and regulatory institutions that are geared toward
the treatment and prevention of disease, not toward enhancement.
There is every reason to believe that morally sound and effective
responses to it will have an institutional component. For one thing,
individuals, acting without the coordination that institutions provide are
unlikely to have either the knowledge or the power to resist the institutional forces which promote the development and use of enhancements.
If this is so, then we should begin to try to move from the exchange of
pros and cons to a constructive discussion of how we can cope, institutionally, with the challenges of enhancement. In Chapter Eight I argue
that one of the central problems of justice that enhancement raises will
require a global institutional response, and I explore what such a
response might look like.

Positions on enhancement

The chief division in the literature on enhancement is not between "pro-enhancement" and "anti-enhancement." It is between "anti-enhancement" and "anti-anti-enhancement." By the "anti-enhancement" stance I mean the view that enhancement as such and across the board ought to be avoided. By the "anti-anti-enhancement" stance I mean the view that enhancement is sometimes permissible.

Although, as I have already suggested, it is sometimes hard to determine exactly what their bottom-line conclusion is, harsh critics of enhancement such as Kass, Sandel, and President Bush's Council on Bioethics seem to be opposed to enhancement across the board, not just some enhancements or some enhancements in some circumstances. One reason to think that they are opposed to enhancement across the board is that the types of objections they raise to enhancement seem to be highly general. If the pursuit of enhancement as such betrays a desire for perfection or total mastery, or a failure to appreciate that our good depends on the naturally given, then presumably every effort to enhance will be morally tainted.

Others, such as George Annas and Jürgen Habermas, may not be opposed to enhancements as such, but are unreservedly opposed to all enhancements that involve germline genetic interventions in human beings—changes that can be passed on to the next generation. In contrast, there seem to be no prominent participants in the debate who are accurately described as "pro-enhancement," if this means they endorse enhancement as enthusiastically and as completely as Sandel and Kass reject it. For example, Jonathan Glover, Julian Savulescu, Nicholas Agar, Dan Brock, Nick Bostrom, David DeGrazia, Anders Sandberg, Eric Juengst, Thomas Murray, Bonnie Steinbock, and myself all reject the anti-enhancement view, yet we all have serious reservations about some enhancements in some circumstances. Further, unlike Habermas and Annas, none of this second group of writers advocates a permanent, blanket prohibition on enhancements involving human germline genetic interventions, although all appreciate the risks of this mode of enhancement and none thinks it is permissible at present. So, here is a striking asymmetry in the debate: there are some prominent writers who roundly condemn enhancement, but none who roundly endorse it.

For reasons I have already indicated in my analogy with globalization, I think that neither a "pro-enhancement" nor an "anti-enhancement" stance makes sense. But since there are prominent participants in the enhancement debate who take the "anti-enhancement" stance, I will provide a detailed critique of it. Finding out exactly what is wrong with the anti-enhancement view will also help us to appreciate what is valuable in it. I shall argue that some of the concerns voiced by anti-enhancement writers are serious, once they are stripped of hyperbole, and that a sound response to the challenges of enhancement must take them into account.

The reasonable alternative to the "anti-enhancement" stance is not the "pro-enhancement" stance but rather "anti-anti-enhancement"—the rejection of the admonition to forego enhancement entirely. The "anti-anti-enhancement" view is not monolithic: it includes some who are enthusiastic about a rather wide range of enhancements and some who are much more cautious and skeptical.

The division between "anti-enhancement" and "anti-anti-enhancement" is not the same as that between "conservatives" and liberals." Some "liberal" writers (or at least who would describe themselves as liberal) have strong reservations about enhancement, or even flirt with the "anti-enhancement" stance, because they believe that enhancements will generally only be available to the rich and worry that this will only worsen existing unjust inequalities. They believe this because they assume, rather than argue, that enhancements, or those enhancements that can have a negative impact on justice, will exclusively be market goods, available only according to ability to pay, *and* that they will be so expensive as to be unaffordable to many. In Chapter Two I challenge this assumption, which frames much of the current debate. I argue that whether or not a particular enhancement is treated simply as a market good or instead as a social good to which citizens have entitlements may depend on whether the State comes to regard it as a technology whose wide diffusion would contribute to national productivity. Here a historical perspective is useful: direct state action, in the form of public education, has played a major role in the diffusion of the most powerful cognitive enhancement technology to date, literacy. That cognitive enhancement has not been a purely market good and the fact that basic education has been treated as an entitlement has significantly limited inequalities in access to education that would otherwise have existed. I also argue that whether, or for how long, an enhancement is affordable only to the rich will depend upon a number of factors, some of which are within our control.

Those who adopt the "anti-anti-enhancement" stance—those who disagree with the wholesale rejection of enhancement—do so in part because they find unconvincing various arguments that purport to show that enhancement is immoral as such or always too risky unconvincing. But they are also impressed with the potential benefits of enhancement. In contrast, for those who adopt the "anti-enhancement" stance, the benefits pale in comparison to the risks, in part because they tend to see enhancements solely or chiefly as vanity goods, unseemly efforts to master the human condition or to achieve perfection, or as attempts to gain a competitive advantage for oneself or one's children. In Chapter Two, I challenge this understanding of the value of enhancements by showing how some enhancements, especially those that improve our cognitive capacities and our capacities for cooperation, could, under the right circumstances, provide much broader, more morally respectable benefits.

As I have already noted, those who reject the "anti-enhancement" view, while more appreciative of the potential benefits of enhancement than their opponents, do not deny that there are serious risks. The risks they acknowledge are diverse, including the worsening of social injustices and the risk of unintended bad biological or psychological consequences. But those who reject the "anti-enhancement" position have too often rested content with unsatisfyingly vague acknowledgments of the problem of risk. With a few notable exceptions, they have not offered much more than platitudes—go slow, proceed with caution, constrain the development of enhancements by the demands of distributive justice, etc.—without providing much guidance on *how* to reduce the risks.[25]

In Chapters Six and Eight, I begin to remedy this deficiency in the anti-anti-enhancement position. Chapter Six offers a set of cautionary heuristics for what many regard as the riskiest mode of enhancement, the genetic modification of human embryos. Chapter Eight outlines an institutional proposal for addressing one of the most serious issues of justice—the possibility that highly beneficial enhancements may not become available to the worst off or may do so too slowly, where this would result in a worsening of unjust inequalities.

The idea of the enhancement enterprise

Because I find the "anti-enhancement" view both morally implausible and unrealistic (like saying "no" to globalization) and the "anti-anti-enhancement" view unsatisfyingly vague, it is incumbent on me to propose a better alternative. My proposal is to try to reconfigure the enhancement debate in a more fruitful way by examining the following question: Is it ethically permissible for a reasonably liberal and democratic society to embark on *the enhancement enterprise*? A society embarks on the enhancement enterprise if, through its regular political processes, it (1) allows considerable freedom to individuals and organizations to develop and choose to use enhancement technologies, including biomedical enhancement technologies, and also (2) devotes significant public resources (a) to research that can be expected to result in enhancement technologies, (b) to creating a vigorous and informed public debate about the benefits and risks of such technologies, and (c) to developing effective and morally sensitive policies and institutions for coping with the challenges of enhancement.

A society that engages in the enhancement enterprise recognizes the *legitimacy* of biomedical enhancement, as one mode of enhancement among others, both as a personal aim that individuals may permissibly pursue and as one permissible policy goal among others with which it must compete, through the political process, for public resources. In its public policy, such a society rejects the view that biomedical enhancement as such, either because it is *enhancement*, rather than the treatment or prevention of disease, or because it uses *biomedical* technology or involves biological changes, is off-limits. By recognizing enhancement, including biomedical enhancement, as a legitimate aim, it implicitly rejects the ill-founded, sweeping generalization that the pursuit of enhancement betrays morally unacceptable motivations or bad character.

When a society undertakes the enhancement enterprise it thereby rejects the anti-enhancement position, the view that biomedical enhancements are to be avoided altogether. More positively, it commits itself to developing the moral and institutional resources needed to pursue enhancements responsibly.

The decision to recognize that enhancement is a legitimate aim for individuals and for social policy makes a great deal of difference. It changes the way deliberations about biomedical enhancements are framed. One of the most important framing shifts is that it signals that biomedical enhancement must compete fairly and openly with other legitimate social goals in the process of allocating resources. In contrast, in a society in which biomedical enhancement comes in through the backdoor, piggy-backing on the treatment and prevention of disease, ever-greater amounts of social resources may be devoted to it, but without any opportunity for democratic, scientifically informed decisions about its comparative worth. Regarding biomedical enhancement as legitimate takes the "no enhancements" alternative off the table, so far a social policy is concerned, but in doing so it *increases* our ability to say "no" to particular biomedical enhancements, either by prohibiting their use or by refusing to support their development with public funding.

A final point about the notion of legitimacy is worth making. Regarding biomedical enhancement as a legitimate social aim does not imply that all individuals are expected to agree that it *is* an appropriate aim for social policy, much less that all must regard it as something they ought to undertake for themselves or their children. In any pluralistic society, there will be some legitimate social policy aims that are rejected by some citizens. Engaging in the enhancement enterprise, as I said earlier, means giving individuals considerable freedom to pursue enhancements if they choose, but also to *not* do so. At some point, however, the implementation of a social policy aimed at achieving widespread use of a particular biomedical enhancement may come into conflict with some individuals' beliefs about what ethical procreation or parenting is or with their own personal preferences about how they ought to act. This is nothing new, of course: educational policies and policies regarding medical care for children also conflict with parental preferences and values.

In my judgment, it will probably be quite a long time before we have biomedical enhancements that would be both powerful enough and safe enough for it to make sense to develop social policies to try to ensure their large-scale implementation. For the foreseeable future, pursuing the enhancement enterprise will largely consist of trying to make good decisions about how much resources ought to be devoted to research on various types of enhancements, how such research can be conducted safely and ethically, and on how to regulate and monitor the effects of enhancements that are being used, either as spin-offs from treatment and prevention of disease or explicitly as enhancements.

One aim of this volume is to try to determine whether the most serious worries about biomedical enhancement—even if they are insufficient to rule out enhancement across the board—give us good reason to refrain from embarking on the enhancement enterprise. My answer will be: no, not at present anyway. But I also hope to make the case for a more positive claim: there are powerful reasons in favor of a society like ours embarking on the enhancement enterprise, and no objections to enhancement that are sufficient to outweigh them, at least at the present time.   *— in favor of means "pro"*

The reasons in favor of the enhancement enterprise are manifold. First, once we get beyond the dubious assumptions that enhancements will be predominantly zero-sum, competitive goods, or expressions of bad character, it becomes clear that the potential social benefits of pursuing the enhancement enterprise are great. Second, the risks of living in a society in which enhancements continue to come in through the backdoor, as new applications of treatment technologies, or through research conducted in countries with inadequate controls on human experimentation, are unacceptably high, given the alternative of pursuing the enhancement enterprise. A third advantage of pursuing the enhancement enterprise is that doing so would facilitate institutional efforts to control enhancements in the name of justice, such as a proposal for a modification of intellectual property rights I explore in Chapter Eight. Fourth, recognizing the legitimacy of enhancement avoids inappropriate medicalization: once we recognize the legitimacy of enhancement as a familiar and admirable human activity, there is no need to pretend that biomedical interventions to achieve enhancement are treatments of diseases, thereby reducing the tendency to multiply diseases and disorders without good reason for doing so. At present, to get (legal) access to cognitive enhancement drugs, individuals must convince physicians (and perhaps themselves as well) that they have attention deficit disorder, narcolepsy, Alzheimer's dementia, or some other cognitive disorder. There is much to be said for being in a society in which efforts to improve our capacities do not require us to view every gap between the way we are now and the way we desire to be as evidence of disease. In a society in which enhancement was recognized as a legitimate human endeavor, there would be less risk of inappropriate *pathologization*.[26] Recognizing the legitimacy of enhancement would liberate not only individuals, but also the research enterprise from the constraints of the medicalization/pathologization framework. The current regulatory framework for drug testing and approval is geared towards showing efficacy in the treatment of disease. Regulation for safety is needed, whether for enhancements or treatments, but shoehorning enhancements into the disease treatment regulatory framework is likely to increase the cost to the consumer and deter some potential researchers and producers.

Consider the case of drugs now being used for cognitive enhancement. Where enhancement is not recognized as legitimate, those with the money to pay black-market prices or the social connections and education to persuade physicians to prescribe Ritalin or other drugs "off label" will have access; others will not. Ironically, prohibiting enhancements out of fear that they will only be available to the rich may exacerbate the problem of injustice. In a society in which the legitimacy of enhancement is recognized, new regulatory institutions can be developed to facilitate the wider and more rapid diffusion of highly beneficial and safe enhancements, in part by eliminating the misplaced constraints of the pathologicalization model and the unnecessary costs they entail.[27]

Agree (margin note)

How to proceed

I have suggested that we ought to get beyond the pros and cons of enhancement and do the hard work of thinking how we can best respond, as individuals and institutionally, to the complex phenomena of enhancement. If that is the case, then why not devote the whole volume to such practical responses?

The reason is simple: before we can go very far in developing appropriate practical responses to the challenges of enhancement, we need to achieve greater clarity on what the real ethical issues are. To do this, we must first debunk the murky rhetoric and replace it with arguments that we can evaluate critically, stop acting as if evolutionary biology is irrelevant to the enhancement debate, face up to the fact that the history of attempts to solve substantive ethical issues by appealing to human nature is a story of unmitigated failures, and try to be more methodologically self-conscious, where this means recognizing when a conclusion depends on reliable empirical evidence and shouldering the responsibility for providing it. In brief, we need to do a better job of *framing* the ethical issues. That is my primary goal in this volume.

Just interesting to think about (margin note)

Love this intention & idea (handwritten note)

From what I have said so far, the reader might conclude that I think there is little of value in the enhancement literature. That is not the case. There is much to be admired. In what follows I hope both to acknowledge the best work on the topic and to build on it. I also believe, however, that this volume will go some distance toward remedying the deficiencies of the current debate listed above, and that if it does it will make a significant new contribution.

My approach to the ethics of enhancement is distinctive in several respects. First, thanks to the generous instruction of three philosophers of biology, David Crawford, Russell Powell, and Alex Rosenberg, it is more informed by an accurate understanding of evolutionary biology.

The second distinctive feature of my approach is the traction that is provided by examining the question of whether a reasonably liberal and democratic society may—or even ought to—embark on the enhancement enterprise. Keeping this question in mind will force us to keep repeating the query: "So what?" or, a bit more respectfully, "What does your argument ("for" or "against" enhancement) imply about what we should or shouldn't do—what's the bottom line?" The question of whether a society like ours may or should (provisionally) pursue the enhancement enterprise is the right question to ask, given that we will have enhancements no matter what any ethicist says and regardless of what political decisions are taken on enhancement. Instead of merely noting the various considerations in favor of or against enhancement, it is more fruitful to try to focus the debate by asking whether these pros and cons can support an answer to the question of whether we ought to undertake the enhancement enterprise.

Third, I believe that my approach is also more methodologically self-conscious than most contributions to the enhancement debate. I make a serious effort to ask when a claim is empirical and when it is conceptual, and if it is the former, whether there is good evidence to support it. I try to avoid reliance on unsupported, *a priori* psychological generalizations.

The majority of my examples of deficiencies in the enhancement debate have been drawn from those who hold "anti-enhancement" views. From this one might infer that I am "pro-enhancement." Not so: I would put myself in the "anti-anti-enhancement" category. But I do want to say something more substantive and action-guiding than the claim that enhancement is sometimes permissible. Focusing on the question of the enhancement enterprise, which I conceive of in

[handwritten margin note:] I do like this way of looking & thinking about things

[handwritten margin note:] I admire this & would like to make an effort to do so in all of my arguments

institutional terms, and exploring a concrete institutional response to problems of justice, will help to achieve this goal. Thus, my approach is distinctive in a fourth and final way: it takes institutions seriously. To put the same point a bit differently: I operate as a political philosopher who recognizes the relevance for ethics of institutional design in the real world.   ⮑ love this, just wondering if institutions ever actually take

This volume does not purport to be a comprehensive treatment of the ethics of biomedical enhancement. I doubt that anyone could do that in ethics a volume of reasonable length; but I am certain that I could not do it into even if given unlimited space. Instead, my aim is to improve the consideration enhancement debate, not to end it, by clearing obstacles from the path themselves of progress and taking a few steps in the right direction. It is worth being if not more explicit about what I will not address in this volume. To do this, it what's is necessary to attempt an outline of a more comprehensive picture of the the point?? ethics of enhancement.

Sorting out the issues

The most important concerns about enhancement fall under eight headings: (1) character, (2) human nature and the natural, (3) the possibility that enhancements would produce beings with a higher moral status than persons, (4) unintended (bad) consequences, (5) justice, (6) research on enhancements, (7) abuses of enhancement technologies by governments (e.g., for unacceptable military applications or suppression of domestic dissent), and (8) the risk of a "new eugenics." My focus is on the first five topics. It is not that I think the other topics are unimportant. I do think, however, that there is something to be said for concentrating on the first five, because unless considerable progress is made on them, one will lack essential resources for fruitfully exploring the last three. For example, how much risk to experimental subjects is permissible will depend, *inter alia*, on how valuable the enhancements one is trying to develop are. Further, if the enhancements in question are ethically impermissible, then presumably research to develop them would be impermissible as well. Similarly, if the benefits of certain enhancements are great enough (and there are no valid moral objections to trying to achieve them), then it may be reasonable to accept a somewhat higher risk that they will be misused by government than would otherwise be the case.

The risk of a "new eugenics," is really two distinct concerns. The first is fear of a resurgence of *state-driven coercive* eugenics: discriminatory, and grossly unjust government policies such as compulsory sterilization, augmented by powerful technologies that the eugenicists only dreamed of, including genetic interventions in human embryos. The second is the worry that even if there is no state-driven eugenics, there will a "laissez-faire eugenics": private choices in a market for enhancements will lead to the same attitudes and results that characterized the old, state-driven eugenics. Most participants in the academic debate about enhancement appear to believe that the risk of a new state-driven eugenics is relatively low, at least in democratic countries with well-entrenched civil and political rights, including reproductive rights. They assume that the rights culture in such countries is sufficiently developed and stable enough—and the "lesson" of the old eugenics sufficiently vivid—that a new state-driven eugenics is unlikely.[28] They focus, instead, on the ethical issues that will arise if enhancements are largely treated as market goods. I have already said why I think this line of thinking is dubious and may lull us into an unwarranted complacency: the state may take an interest in the development and diffusion of those enhancements that promise greater productivity. To that extent, I address the concern about a new state-driven eugenics and take it *more seriously* than is usually the case. One point I make in this regard is worth previewing: in the case of enhancements that promise increased productivity, the worry, at least in states with a deeply rooted "rights culture," may not be *coercive* state action (compulsory sterilization or compulsory genetic selection or engineering of human embryos), but rather state subsidies for and encouragement of individual's choices to undertake enhancements.

Such a "softer," noncoercive state-driven eugenics would build upon other forces that encourage recourse to enhancements. The combination of state encouragement, vigorous private marketing, and the herd-like impetus of popular culture might result in a situation in which individuals had more choices, but were worse off. For example, even if the state did not force people to use technologies to produce "better" embryos, many people might feel compelled to do so, in the face of government subsidies and social pressure to avoid having "substandard" offspring.

Such concerns clearly should not be dismissed, but it is important to recognize that they are extremely speculative. At present we simply don't

know enough either about how the state will regard various enhancements or whether individual values and social norms will develop in such
a way as to exacerbate or mitigate dangerous state policies regarding
enhancement. It is safe to say that we should be on the alert for such
developments, but at present the best strategy may be to concentrate on
the first five concerns about enhancement. Working out a reasonable
response to them may well be a necessary step toward mitigating the risk
of a "new eugenics."

feels likely [handwritten annotation]

Why bother with debunking bad arguments and murky rhetoric?

If some of the anti-enhancement "arguments" are as flimsy or confused
as I say they are, why bother with criticizing them? There are two
reasons. First, sometimes there is a valid concern to be extracted from
the verbal thicket (or to be found in its general vicinity). Second, bad
arguments can be quite influential. If the aim of Practical Ethics is to
make things better (or at least to prevent them from getting worse),
morally speaking, then practical ethicists have an obligation to address
bad arguments, if they think they are influential.[29] I will focus special
attention on debunking bad arguments that could be seen as ruling out
embarking on the enhancement enterprise.

Enhancement and well-being

To enhance is to improve, augment, make better. There is considerable
controversy about how exactly to define "biomedical enhancement" in
the way that is most fruitful for exploring the ethical issues. To avoid
wasting space that is better allocated to substantive issues, I will operate
with a relatively uncontroversial definition: a biomedical enhancement is
a deliberate intervention, applying biomedical science, which aims to
improve an existing capacity that most or all normal human beings
typically have, or to create a new capacity, by acting directly on the
body or brain.

that feels icky, just a feeling but not empirical [handwritten annotation]

One advantage of this definition is that it helps us to avoid a simple
mistake: thinking that an enhancement by definition makes one better
off. Enhanced hearing, in a noisy environment, might make an easily
distracted person worse off. Enhanced memory, unless accompanied
by enhanced capacities to control the activation of memories or the
management of their psychological effects, might also be problematic.

The attempt to enhance a capacity can go wrong in at least two ways, then: it can fail to achieve its goal; or it can achieve its goal but make us worse off.

Another advantage of the above definition of biomedical enhancements is that it makes clear the fact that there can be important enhancements that are not biomedical. For example, literacy is an exceedingly powerful cognitive enhancement. Depending on how one looks at what literacy enables us to do, one might say either that it greatly improves the cognitive capacities that humans had before the invention of writing or that it gives us new cognitive capacities. Either way, the point is that literate human beings can perform cognitive tasks that illiterate ones can't and that (some of) these tasks are extremely valuable. Literacy does not count as a *biomedical* enhancement, according to our definition, because teaching people to read and write is not an intervention that applies biomedical science to improve existing capacities by acting directly on the brain or body. As it turns out, learning to read and write *does* change the brain, but that is not the aim of teaching people to read and write and, at least until recently, teaching literacy has not relied on biomedical science. Similarly, institutions tremendously enhance human capacities for cooperation and coordination, but they are not biomedical enhancements.

Literacy and institutions, although not biomedical enhancements, have had profound impacts on the human genome: they have laid the groundwork for developments that have brought together formerly isolated various human populations, allowing genetic combinations that would not otherwise have occurred. The agrarian revolution and the development of cities that it made possible have also changed the human gene pool, by subjecting human beings to diseases that have selected for disease resistant genes. Qua enhancement, what matters is that literacy improves cognitive functioning; the fact that it does so without biomedical interventions is irrelevant to its being an enhancement. Whether cognitive gains are achieved by learning to read and write or by implanting a microchip in the brain is irrelevant; the term "enhancement" is equally applicable to the two cases.

The examples of literacy and institutions illustrate three important points to keep in mind in our exploration of the ethics of biomedical enhancement. First, enhancement is not new. To a large extent, human history is the history of enhancement. Second, at this point in the

even though I don't like the concept, it seems to be valid

development of biomedical science, there is no reason to believe biomedical enhancements will be the most profound or morally problematic enhancements. Every major enhancement has created moral and physical risks. (The awesome collective cognitive enhancement we call science has created the risk of a nuclear holocaust, for example.) Third, some non-biomedical enhancements produce biological effects, including changes in the human genome. So, if biomedical enhancements are morally problematic, it cannot be because they are enhancements or because they raise moral issues or because they involve biological or genetic effects.

Types and modes of enhancement

Five types of enhancement are widely discussed in the literature on the ethics of biomedical enhancement: improvements in physical characteristics such as speed, strength, and endurance; improvements in cognitive capacities, such as various aspects of memory, information-processing, and reasoning; improvements in affect, emotion, motivation, or temperament; improvements in immunity or resistance to diseases; and increased longevity. In principle, each of these types of enhancement could be achieved by a plurality of *modes* of enhancement—different biomedical means for bringing the desired improvement about.

The number of modes of biomedical enhancement is increasing as biomedical science rapidly advances. It would be unwise, therefore, to try to provide an exhaustive list. Instead, I will simply indicate what some of the more promising existing or realistically anticipated modes of biomedical interventions are ones that can reasonably be expected to be harnessed for the pursuit of some or all of the types of enhancement listed above. These include (1) selection of embryos for implantation according to genotype (if genotypes associated with "better than normal" phenotypes could be reliably identified); (2) genetic engineering of embryos, by insertion of human or nonhuman animal genes or artificial chromosomes; (3) administration of drugs (e.g., cognitive enhancement drugs); (4) implantation of genetically engineered tissue or organs; and (5) brain–computer interface technologies, using nanotechnology to connect neural tissue with electronic circuits.

With the possible exception of genetic engineering of embryos, it is hard to discern any morally relevant differences among these different biomedical modes of enhancement. It is interesting to note that for the most part the concerns about enhancement apply, not just across a wide variety of modes of biomedical enhancement, but to nonbiomedical enhancements as well. In fact, as I have already noted, the harshest criticisms of biomedical enhancement appear to apply to enhancements *per se*, whether biomedical or not. This striking generality ought to make us wary of what I described earlier as the anti-enhancement position— the rejection of biomedical enhancements as such—because it means that if we accept that view, we would not only have to reject cognitive enhancement drugs, but must also regard literacy, institutions, and the agrarian revolution in a highly unfavorable light as well.

To appreciate this point, let us focus for a moment on literacy. The spread of literacy and its integration into the fabric of our lives undoubtedly has made serious encroachments on the domain of "the unbidden" or "the given," such as by introducing a higher degree of coordination and predictability in human affairs, and by enabling the development of science that can be used to control and shape many aspects of our environment, including medical treatments that significantly reduce uncertainties regarding health and illness. I, for one, am *grateful* (to our ancestors) that appreciation of "the given" or "openness to the unbidden" did not prevent them from developing this powerful cognitive enhancement.

Some participants in the enhancement debate have tried to rely on a distinction between therapy (understood broadly as including the treatment and prevention of disease) and enhancement. There are some contexts in which the distinction can be clearly drawn, and some in which the line is blurry. The chief point, however, is that when the distinction can be drawn it is of limited if any use from the standpoint of moral guidance. The mere fact that an intervention is an enhancement rather than a therapy does nothing to show that it is impermissible, or even morally problematic. Numeracy, literacy, and computers are all cognitive enhancements, but that doesn't count against them at all, morally speaking. Some biomedical enhancements, perhaps many, may turn out to be no more morally problematic than these historical enhancements. Of course, there may be moral objections to the use of cognitive enhancement drugs in certain contexts or for certain purposes; but it is not the fact that they enhance normal cognitive performance rather than treat or prevent disease that makes them problematic. After all, caffeine is a cognitive enhancement drug, but it would be unreasonable to say that people should be able to get access to it only if they have a prescription and suffer from a disease, such as narcolepsy.

On some accounts, "the ends of medicine" are restricted to treating and preventing disease, restoring normal functioning, and offering comfort and care for those who are ill or disabled. Talk about the "ends of medicine" is essentialist talk and as such it ought to be regarded with a good deal of skepticism, especially when applied to medicine. As I show in Chapter Two, essentialist talk often disguises highly controversial moral claims as factual claims and this is hardly conducive to fruitful ethical analysis. Instead of contending that medicine *is* this or is that, we should be asking whether we should have this or that sort of institution or this or that sort of profession, no matter what we call it. It might turn out that there is something to be said for having an institution or a profession that we call medicine and that focuses on treatment, prevention, restoration of normal functioning, comfort, and care, rather than on enhancement. That is perfectly compatible, however, with also saying that we should recognize different professional roles that encompass the provision of enhancement. The key point is that even if one accepts the controversial view that enhancement is not a "proper" end of medicine, that tells us nothing about whether enhancement is morally permissible. Nor does it even exclude the medical profession from playing an important role in the enhancement enterprise. Whether or not biomedical enhancement is regarded as being part of medicine, medical expertise will be needed to assess its safety and monitor its effects, during the course of research and when the technology is deployed.

In my reflections on biomedical enhancement, I will not spend much time on the enhancement/therapy distinction. Instead, I will meet the critics of enhancement on their own terms, arguing that even if certain biomedical interventions are clearly enhancements and not therapies, this fact about them is of no moral significance and that they must be assessed on other grounds.

In much of this volume, I will concentrate on enhancement drugs more than on other modes of biomedical enhancement, for two reasons. First, pharmaceutical enhancements are on the way, if not already here. On some accounts, performance-enhancing drugs, if they have not already done so, will before long extend the upper bound of normal human physical strength, speed, and stamina. Several widely available drugs, including Ritalin, Adderall, and Provigil, improve cognitive functioning in normal individuals, and there is reason to expect that much more powerful cognitive enhancement drugs will soon be developed. Focusing on enhancement drugs, rather than on more exotic interventions such as nanotechnology-enabled microcomputer brain implants reduces the risk of exceeding the bounds of reasonable speculation. Second, pharmaceutical enhancements are likely to be less expensive (especially after the drugs go "off patent") than other modes of biomedical enhancement, so focusing on them increases the likelihood of engaging issues that will be important to many people.

The plan of this volume

The present chapter sketches the landscape of the enhancement debate, identifies its deficiencies, and previews my efforts to improve the quality of the debate. Chapter Two places biomedical enhancements squarely in the context of a long history of enhancements and argues that it is illuminating to view the ethics of enhancement through the lens of the *ethics of development*. ("Development" here is used in the economists' sense, not as in texts on the biological development of individual organisms, i.e., ontogeny.) The key to achieving this framing shift is to recognize that some enhancements—especially those that improve cognition—should not be seen solely, or even primarily, as zero-sum. This chapter then goes on to make the case for the plausibility of the proposal that in a reasonably liberal and democratic society it is morally permissible to pursue the enhancement enterprise. The same reasons that support the conclusion that embarking (provisionally) on the enhancement enterprise is morally permissible also do a good deal to support the stronger conclusion that it is ethically obligatory to do so.

Chapter Three articulates and evaluates the claim that the pursuit of enhancement is an expression of defective character, or in more traditional terms, a symptom of vice or at least of the lack of virtue. I argue that once we puncture the inflated rhetoric, serious concerns remain, but that they do not support anything approaching a blanket rejection of biomedical enhancement—not even in the case of what some regard as the most radical biomedical enhancement of all, the genetic engineering of human embryos. Nor do they amount to a cogent case against pursuing the enhancement enterprise.

Chapter Four examines a cluster of worries about enhancement that are framed in terms of human nature or the natural. The chief conclusion of this chapter is that appeals to human nature and the natural cannot illuminate the most difficult issues concerning biomedical enhancement, that anything of value that can be framed in these terms can be better framed without recourse to them, and that they are so confused that we should avoid them altogether in grappling with the ethical issues of enhancement.

Chapter Five explores the possibility that the mainstream of traditional Conservative thought in the tradition of Edmund Burke provides a better vantage point from which to argue against the enhancement project than the work of contemporary conservative bioethicists such as Fukuyama, Sandel, and Kass. I conclude that mainstream traditional Conservative thought provides no conclusive reasons against pursuing the enhancement project and—surprisingly—supplies a powerful reason *in favor* of pursuing it. A central Conservative thesis is that human nature includes cognitive imperfections that doom efforts to achieve large-scale improvements in the human condition. I argue that this central conservative thesis speaks strongly in favor of enhancement, if these cognitive imperfections may be safely ameliorated through the use of biotechnologies. I also argue that, at present, there is no good reason to conclude that our cognitive imperfections are so severe as to rule out our significantly ameliorating them.

Chapter Six grapples with what I believe to be the most serious objection to embarking on the enhancement project: the risk of unintended bad consequences. Here I argue that the discussion of this risk has been distorted by a failure to appreciate the full range of the possible benefits of enhancement and by mistaken views about evolution. The simple but often neglected point here is that the assessment of risk is comparative. Building on the discussion of the potential benefits of enhancement in Chapter Two and on the basis of a more adequate understanding of evolution, I offer a set of cautionary heuristics that are designed to reduce the risk of unintended bad consequences in the case of what many regard as the riskiest type of enhancement: deliberate germline genetic modification.

Chapter Seven addresses a cluster of concerns that revolve around a fundamental, but obscure concept that lies at the heart of moral theory: moral status. I distinguish between the claim that biomedical enhancements could eventually produce posthumans (beings of a different species from *Homo sapiens*) and the quite different claim that they could produce postpersons—beings with a higher status than that of persons. I also argue that the concern that enhancements may render the concept of human rights obsolete have either failed to distinguish between posthumans and postpersons or misunderstood what human rights are. Finally, I argue that even if there is little risk that enhancement will produce a morally bifurcated world of persons and postpersons, it could produce challenges to equality that cut deeper than the familiar worry about exacerbating existing unjust distributions of resources.

Chapter Eight continues the exploration of justice issues, focusing on the problem of inadequate diffusion: the worry that valuable biomedical enhancements may not be available or may only be available after an extended period of time, to the world's poorest people. In keeping with Chapter One's emphasis on the fact that enhancement is not new and that biomedical enhancement is not distinctively morally problematic, I situate this problem as one aspect of a larger problem of inadequate diffusion of beneficial technologies, and offer a global institutional response to this larger problem. Thus, the volume concludes with an example of how to move beyond the exchange of pros and cons to a constructive, practical, institutional response to one of the major challenges of biomedical enhancement.

Beyond humanity?

The question posed by the title of this volume is deliberately ambiguous. On one interpretation, the question is whether biomedical technologies will enable us to go beyond humanity in the sense of overcoming limitations that human beings have always had to live with and that may be included in a reasonable concept of what it is to be human.

On a second interpretation, the title poses the question of whether enhancement is overreach: Does humanity, as it is now, have the wisdom and the character to face the challenges of enhancement, or is responsible enhancement beyond our human capacities? Both of these questions, I shall argue, are even more complex and more difficult to answer than they appear to be.

Yes

b/c we are
selfish & greedy —this has
been proven!

Notes

1. The quoted passage combines common anti-enhancement views, each of which I carefully articulate, reference, and analyze as the argument of this book progresses.
2. See, for example, Michael Sandel (2007), *The Case Against Perfection: Ethics in the Age of Genetic Engineering* (Harvard University Press), pp. 99–100. Sandel suggests that "there is something appealing, even intoxicating, about a vision of human freedom unfettered by the given." But he contends that our quest for mastery is flawed because it "threatens to banish our appreciation of life as a gift, and to leave us with nothing to affirm or behold outside our own will." Ibid.
3. President's Council on Bioethics (2003), *Human Cloning and Human Dignity: An Ethical Inquiry* (Washington, DC: National Bioethics Advisory Commission), pp. 287–290; Sandel 2007, supra note 2.
4. Michael Sandel (2004), "The Case Against Perfection: What's Wrong With Designer Children, Bionic Athletes, and Genetic Engineering?" *The Atlantic Monthly* 292(3): 51–62; Michael Sandel (2007), *The Case Against Perfection: Ethics in the Age of Genetic Engineering* (Cambridge, MA: Harvard University Press) pp. 93–95.
5. Many philosophers of biology not only reject the natural-unnatural distinction (see Marc Ereshefsky (2007), "Where the Wild Things Are: Environmental Preservation and Human Nature," *Biology and Philosophy* 22: 57–72), but also the notion of 'normal function', where the latter is not simply a statistical generalization, but rather a normatively infused one. See David Hull (1986), "On Human Nature," in *Philosophy of Science Association*, vol. 2(A), Fine and P. Machamer (eds.) (East Lansing, MI: Philosophy of Science Association) pp. 3–13.
6. Jürgen Habermas (2003), *The Future of Human Nature* (Cambridge: Polity).
7. See Francis Fukuyama (2003), *Our Posthuman Future: Consequences of the Biotechnology Revolution* (Profile Books). Fukuyama views genetic enhancement technologies as a threat to human nature. He states (p. 172) as follows: "What is it that we want to protect from any future advances in biotechnology? The answer is, we want to protect the full range of complex, evolved natures against attempts at self-modification. We do not want to disrupt either the unity or the continuity of human nature, and thereby the human rights that are based on it." See also George Annas (1998), "Why we should ban human cloning," *New England Journal of Medicine* 339: 122–125; Leon Kass (1997), "The Wisdom of Repugnance," *New Republic* 216(22): 17–26.
8. Allen Buchanan (2009), "Human Nature and Enhancement," *Bioethics* 23(3): 141–150; see also Hull 1986, surpa note 5.
9. For exceptions, see R. Powell (forthcoming), "The Evolutionary Biological Implications of Human Genetic Engineering," *Journal of Medicine and Philosophy*; R. Powell, and A. Buchanan (2009), "Breaking Evolution's

32   *The Landscape of the Enhancement Debate*

Chains: The Promise of Enhancement by Design," in *Enhancing Human Capacities*, Julian Savulescu (ed.) (Oxford University Press); N. Bostrom and A. Sandberg (2009), "The Wisdom of Nature: An Evolutionary Heuristic for Human Enhancement" in *Human Enhancement*, Julian Savulescu and Nick Bostrom (eds.) (Oxford University Press).

10. For a discussion, see Norman Daniels (2009), "Can Anyone Really Be Talking About Modifying Human Nature," in *Human Enhancement*, Julian Savulescu and Nick Bostrom (eds.) (Oxford University Press), pp. 25–42.

11. See Matt Ridley (2003), *Nature Via Nurture: Genes, Experience, and What Makes Us Human* (New York: Harper Collins). The idea that there are traits whose development does not depend on the environment was completely undermined by the middle of the twentieth century, when it was shown that environmental variables are indispensable for the development of nearly all phenotypic traits. See D. Lehrman, "A critique of Konrad Lorenz's theory of instinctive behavior." *The Quarterly Review of Biology*, 28 (1953): 337–363.

12. See, for example, Peter Richerson and Robert Boyd (2005), *Not By Genes Alone: How Culture Transformed Human Evolution* (Chicago, IL: University of Chicago Press).

13. See Thomas Murray (2007), 'Enhancement', in the *Oxford Handbook of Bioethics*, B. Steinbock (ed.) pp. 491–515 (Oxford University Press); Allen Buchanan (2009), 'Human Nature and Enhancement,' *Bioethics* 23(3): 141–150; Bonnie Steinbock (2008), 'Designer babies: choosing our children's genes', *Lancet* 372(9646): 1294–1295.

14. Cited in Richard Dawkins (2003), *A Devil's Chaplain: Reflections on Hope, Lies, Science, and Love* (Houghton Mifflin Harcourt) p. 8.

15. Sandel 2007, supra note 2. See also Leon Kass (2003), "Ageless Bodies, Happy Souls," *The New Atlantis* 1: 9–28; Leon Kass (2004), "L'Chaim and Its Limits: Why Not Immortality?" in *The fountain of Youth: Cultural, Scientific, and Ethical Perspectives on a Biomedical Goal*, Stephen Post and Robert Benstock (eds.) (Oxford University Press).

16. Sandel 2007, supra note 2, pp. 99–100.

17. See, for example, Michael Sandel (2007) *The Case Against Perfection: Ethics in the Age of Genetic Engineering* (Cambridge, MA: Harvard University Press) pp. 89–92.

18. Leon Kass, "Ageless Bodies, Happy Souls," *The New Atlantis* 1 (2003): 9–28.

19. It may be worth noting here that some of the world's major religions teach that it is a good thing to want immortality.

20. See President's Council on Bioethics 2003, supra note 3, pp. 101–106; Kass 1997, supra note 7.

21. See President's Council on Bioethics 2003, supra note 3, pp. 110–112.

22. Michael Sandel (2007), *The Case Against Perfection: Ethics in the Age of Genetic Engineering* (Harvard University Press), p. 96.

23. I characterize the point that the enhancement debate should take character into account as uncontroversial for two reasons. First, it is so obviously plausible as to be a truism. Second, contrary to what Sandel suggests, the debate has recognized that character is relevant for quite a long time. For example, at least since 2000 there has been a vigorous discussion in the scholarly literature as to whether biomedical enhancements of the characteristics of children expresses morally deficient attitudes toward people with disability. See Dan Brock (1995), "'The Non-Identity Problem and Genetic Harms—The Case of Wrongful Handicaps," *Bioethics* 9(3): 269–275.

24. Jonathan Glover, *Choosing Children: Genes, Design, and Disability* (Oxford: Oxford University Press, 2003, p. 36).

25. See, for example, Julian Savulescu, who simply replies to the worry that enhancements might bring discrimination toward the unenhanced that "Discrimination is our choice—not written into our biology." Julian Savulescu (2006), "Justice, Fairness, and Enhancement," *Annals of the New York Academy of Sciences* 1093(1): 321–338. The question is this: how are we to make this choice effective?

26. See Anders Sandberg (forthcoming), "The Economics of Cognitive Development," in *Enhancing Human Capabilities*, Julian Savulescu *et al.* (eds.) (Oxford: Wiley-Blackwell).

27. Greely, Henry, Sahakian, Barbara, Harris, John, Kessler, Ronald C., Gazzaniga, Michael, Campbell, Philip, Farah, and Martha J. (2008). "Towards responsible use of cognitive-enhancing drugs by the healthy." *Nature* 456: 702–705.

28. Nicholas Agar (2004), *Liberal Eugenics: In Defence of Human Enhancement* (Wiley-Blackwell).

29. Allen Buchanan (2009), "Philosophy and Public Policy: A Role for Social Moral Epistemology." *Journal of Applied Philosophy* 26(3): 276–290.

CHAPTER TWO

Enhancement and Human Development

I have four aims in this chapter: (1) to begin to clear a path for more fruitful thinking about the ethics of enhancement by exposing two false framing assumptions that have seriously distorted the debate; (2) to demystify the topic by showing that enhancement is not new, but instead is a fundamental theme in human history; (3) to say enough about the character and the magnitude of potential benefits of biomedical enhancements to begin to put concerns about the risks of enhancement in proper perspective; and (4) to make a provisional case for what I referred to in Chapter One as *the enhancement enterprise*. By a provisional case I mean a *pro tanto* case—an argument for pursuing the enhancement enterprise for now.

Each of the subsequent chapters of this volume examines worries about enhancement that might be thought to defeat the provisional case for the enhancement enterprise. By the end of the volume, I hope to have shown that concerns about enhancement, properly understood, provide valuable guidance for *how* we should pursue the enhancement enterprise, but *not* good reasons for refraining from it.

Two framing assumptions that distort the debate

The first framing assumption is that the most significant benefits are *private* or *personal goods*, that is, advantages to the persons who are enhanced (or to their parents in the case of enhanced children). Call this the Personal Goods Assumption. Some writers who subscribe to this first assumption also hold that the risks of enhancement include not only harms to individuals but also social or collective harms, from the destruction of "(truly) human reproduction"[1] or the loss of the sense of "giftedness,"[2] to an exacerbation of existing unjust inequalities,[3] to the loss of our species' fitness for survival.[4] Each of these predicted harms affects individuals directly, but those who warn of these harms also emphasize their social or collective dimension. They worry that a society in which biomedical enhancements are pursued on a large scale would be a bad or unhealthy society, with distorted values and relationships.

Critics of enhancement also focus on the exercise of choice and the satisfaction of aesthetic tastes or preferences to excel in competition.[5] They paint an unflattering picture of the benefits of enhancement and the motives that prompt people to undertake them. In addition, there is a tendency to concentrate on cases where the enhancement of some will disadvantage those who are not enhanced—to assume that enhancement is a zero sum affair.[6] Proponents of enhancement often lend credibility to the assumption that the benefits of enhancement will primarily if not exclusively accrue to those who have them by assuming that there will be a free market for enhancements, where access will depend on ability to pay.

According to this first framing assumption, the key public policy decision is whether the private benefits that enhancements would confer are worth the risk of social harms that they may produce. This way of framing the debate gives short shrift to the possibility that enhancements might bring significant social benefits.[7]

I will argue that the Personal Goods Assumption is false because some enhancements, including those that are most likely to garner the re-sources needed to make them widespread, will have the potential to bring broad social benefits that cannot be reduced to the gains for those who are enhanced (or their parents). I will also argue that it is mistaken to focus on situations in which enhancements will have zero sum effects. My critique of the first framing assumption will rest on two key theses: (a) that some enhancements will increase human productivity broadly conceived and thereby create the potential for large-scale increases in human well-being, and (b) that the enhancements that are most likely to attract sufficient resources to become widespread will be those that promise increased productivity and will often exhibit what economists call *network effects*: the benefit to an individual of being enhanced will depend upon, or at least be greatly augmented by others having the enhancement as well. When these two points are appreciated, it becomes clear that we must take the potential social benefits of enhancements—and hence *the social costs of forgoing* enhancements—very seriously.

Once we attend to the productivity–increasing effects of enhancements and their network effects, it becomes clear how misleading it is to think of enhancements as zero sum. I will argue, then, that the Personal Goods Assumption is not only false, but pernicious, because it skews the debate toward the rejection of enhancement by overlooking some of the most powerful reasons for enhancement.

The second framing assumption is that because of the near universal condemnation of eugenics, enhancements will be market goods, a matter of personal choice, not state action, at least in liberal societies.[8] Call this the Market Goods Assumption. When combined with the Personal Goods Assumption, it implies that *the* key ethical problem, in liberal societies, is that of avoiding or ameliorating the social harms that are likely to result from the pursuit of enhancements by individuals in a market for enhancements.

My critique of the first framing assumption will show that the second is also false. The argument can be previewed as follows. Historically, governments have shown a keen interest in increasing productivity. They have often invested heavily in education and public health, not out of regard for the good or the rights of individuals, but because they wanted to "build a stronger nation" (in the case of Bismarck's Germany, for example) or to promote "economic growth." Given this historical fact, it is naïve to assume that the state will abstain from encouraging the development and utilization of enhancements that promise significant increases in productivity. And if this is the case, then focusing exclusively on the problem of how to restrain individual choice in a market for enhancement may leave us unprepared to cope with crucial issues regarding the role of the state.

Finally, building on the point that enhancements can increase productivity very broadly construed and thereby have the potential to provide large-scale gains in human well-being, I will suggest a more basic framing shift in how we conceive of the ethics of enhancement: we ought to view it as one important dimension of *the ethics of development*. I will argue that what is misleadingly called the history of economic development (as if it concerned only the development of the economy) is largely the story of human enhancement. My conclusion here will be that participants in the current debate about enhancement either fail to understand that enhancement is an ancient and characteristic human endeavor, or else they mistakenly assume that there is a moral distinction between enhancing human capabilities by the application of biotechnologies and other modes of enhancement.[9]

Human enhancement, productivity, and development

The ubiquity of enhancement

In the broadest and most straightforward sense, to enhance human beings is to expand their capabilities—to enable them to do what normal human beings have hitherto not been able to do. Understood in this way, enhancement is ubiquitous in human history. Literacy and numeracy are among the most impressive human cognitive enhancements to date.[10] Literacy increases our communicative abilities and our ability to commit ourselves to future actions (as in the case of complex planning of actions undertaken with others, written contracts, and treaties). It enables us to understand the past through written records and augments our capacity not just to remember but also to reflect on and find meaning in our experiences. Literacy is at the heart of the scientific enterprise, and the application of science to practical matters has extended our capacity for agency in myriad ways. Taken together, literacy and numeracy are profound and far-reaching cognitive enhancements. Computers, building on the platform of literacy and numeracy, extend human cognitive capacities even farther.[11]

Agriculture was a momentous enhancement. It enabled large numbers of distantly related individuals to live together in one location year-round, which was a necessary condition for a complex and persisting division of labor, including the rise of a class of individuals who do "mental" rather than physical work, and for the emergence of cities and political institutions.[12] When agriculture became efficient enough, it created surpluses that could be exchanged and thereby increased humans' capability for engaging in peaceful relationships with strangers. The agricultural revolution that began in England around 1760 had dramatic positive effects on human physical well-being through better nutrition, which in turn meant greater resistance to disease and greater longevity.[13]

Institutions are remarkable enhancements. They increase our capability for coordinated interactions and hence for achieving the many goods that depend on coordination. They augment the physical and even the moral powers of individuals and groups. Legal systems are a salient example of how institutions can augment our moral powers: they can enable individuals to behave justly toward one another, in part by providing an authoritative specification of rights. By enforcing rules of peaceful interaction, legal institutions also increase our capacity for restraining our aggressive impulses and provide assurance that others will not take advantage of our restraint.

Avoiding biomedical enhancement exceptionalism

It would be a mistake to object that the foregoing accomplishments are not enhancements in the sense relevant to the current debate because they are merely *external* or *environmental* changes rather than changes *in us* and hence do not qualify as the enhancement of human beings. The better nutrition provided by the agricultural revolution of the mid-eighteenth century significantly changed human beings' bodies by overcoming the stunting effects of under-nutrition, and altered their minds by facilitating neurological development. In addition, there is evidence that literacy actually changes the brain.[14] External or environmental innovations can change us profoundly.

[Although computers are external to our bodies, it would also be a mistake to say that computers are not really enhancements, not improvements of normal human cognitive capabilities. Computers overcome many of the biological limitations of the human brain's information processing and calculating functions, improving our cognitive powers in a perfectly straightforward sense. Similarly, the ability to engage in coordinated activities with large numbers of others made possible by institutions, and the myriad cultural developments based on numeracy, literacy, and science, have helped make us who we are. They have profoundly changed our conception of ourselves and our world and shaped our most basic social relations. To call the great historical enhancements merely external or environmental is tantamount to denying that culture plays a significant role in our individual and collective identities, and it overlooks the indispensable role that culture plays in the development of basic human capacities.

Compared to the great historical enhancements, the changes that are likely to be brought about by biomedical enhancements, including germline interventions to increase intelligence or physical strength or longevity, *might* turn out to be rather puny. At the very least, the comparison debunks the common assumption that biomedical enhancements are inherently more profound and for that reason more morally problematic.

Whether an enhancement involves a direct and deliberate modification of the human body does not seem to be of any moral significance in itself. Because of past enhancements, we are born into a world in which literacy is a prominent feature of life for most people, in which tens of millions of people have computers, and in which social interaction increasingly occurs in institutionally structured environments that extend far beyond the boundaries of kinship groups. These enhancements surely affect our lives more deeply than would the routine implantation of tiny computers or genetically engineered tissue in our brains to increase the speed of our neural processing, or the insertion of genes in embryos to provide resistance to infectious diseases.

The changes that the great historical enhancements have wrought are not only internal in the sense that they are changes in us, improvements in *our* capabilities, not merely modifications of our environment or artifacts that are external to us; they are also, for practical purposes, *irreversible.* Given how much we benefit from literacy and numeracy and how foundational these cognitive enhancements are in modern society, any attempt to abandon them would surely fail, not in the least because of familiar barriers to the collective action that would be required for such an astonishing project. Retreating to a hunting and gathering mode of existence would require a vast reduction in the human population, not to mention the loss of all the human goods that depend upon agriculture. Thus it is quite misleading to say that it is only now, in the age of molecular biology, that human beings are able to change themselves irreversibly.

In fact, in some cases it is much easier to reverse biomedical enhancements than cultural enhancements. For example, we already know how to block the expression of genes that have been inserted into laboratory animals and to make genetic changes that have to be switched on by the administration of a drug if they are to produce a change in phenotype. When a biomedical enhancement has to be sustained by the administration of a drug, reversing the enhancement is achieved simply by ceasing to take the drug. So, if there is a moral difference between biomedical enhancements and the traditional enhancements that have come about through cultural change, it is not that the former are irreversible.

Further, merely to observe that the great historical enhancements have affected the biology of human beings is to underestimate their effects on our biology. They have also contributed to the evolution of the human genome. For instance, the proliferation of dairy farming in Middle Eastern and European populations created selection pressures that led to the evolution of genes associated with lactose tolerance.[15] The most obvious effect on the human genome is that human beings are surviving to reproduce who otherwise would not; to that extent the great historical enhancements have contributed to greater genetic diversity in our species. In addition, technologies of transportation have facilitated the mingling of gene pools that were previously isolated. Finally, the great historical enhancements have led to concentrations of populations that have facilitated epidemics, which in turn have selected for disease-resistant genotypes. In other words, the historical enhancements have changed selective pressures, making some traits that were adaptive now maladaptive, and vice versa. *So, it is simply not true that for the first time human beings are becoming capable of changing their biology; the more accurate statement is that for the first time they are becoming capable of changing their biology deliberately, in accordance with what they value, on the basis of scientific knowledge, rather than haphazardly.*

At this point it might be objected that the momentous historical developments I have listed are not really enhancements because enhancements are improvements of the capabilities that are *normal* for human beings, and that writing, living in large-scale institutions, etc., are all normal for human beings. This objection is implausible. We *now* consider literacy, the use of computers, and the ability to engage in large-scale coordinated, complex activities through the functioning of institutions to be "normal" capabilities for human beings, but for most of the time in which human beings existed they were not. Of course, the great historical enhancements would not have occurred if human beings had not shared certain biological characteristics, but that is a different matter, and, besides, the same is true of biomedical enhancements. The point of pursuing biomedical enhancements is to improve human capabilities, and whether doing this is a good idea or not cannot be settled by arbitrarily defining "enhancement" in a way that excludes the most dramatic and far-reaching improvements of human capabilities that have occurred so far.

Nor would it be plausible to say that the great historical improvements are not enhancements because they do not extend our abilities beyond what is *natural* for human beings.

As we shall see in Chapter Four, the term "natural" is ambiguous, and failure to sort out the different meanings causes much mischief in the enhancement debate. If "natural" here means "in accordance with the laws of nature (that is, not supernatural)," then both the historical improvements in human capabilities and the most radical biomedical enhancements are natural; and on the definition of an enhancement as an improvement beyond what is natural for human beings, *neither* would count as enhancements. If "natural" instead means "fitting or proper," then to say that the historical improvements are natural but that biomedical improvements are not is simply to beg the question of whether there is some morally important intrinsic difference between the two. If "natural" means that which occurs without human intervention, then it is true that biomedical enhancements are not natural, but the same is true of agriculture, medicine, institutions, and much else of what we rightly value. Finally, if "natural" is contrasted with that which involves the use of artifices, that is, tools in the broadest sense, then biomedical enhancements are not natural, but the same is true of the labor-saving and in some cases life-saving devices that we rely on every day.

So, regardless of whether one defines "enhancement" as improvement on normal or natural human abilities (in any of the senses of "natural" noted above), the great historical enhancements I have listed have as much claim to be called enhancements of human beings as biomedical enhancements do. In the next chapter I explore the relevance of the ideas of human nature and the natural for the enhancement debate, arguing that they provide little substantive guidance, tend to confuse the issues, and can be eliminated in favor of other concepts that are less liable to rhetorical abuses.

It is also worth emphasizing that the great historical enhancements have the same morally problematic features that worry critics of biomedical enhancement. Consider two common allegations against biomedical enhancements: that they will foster distributive injustices (because they will only be available to the better-off),[16] and that reliance on them will lead to the atrophy of valuable skills or capacities. Once again, literacy and the development of institutions, two of the most momentous historical enhancements, serve to illustrate the point. When literacy was the possession of the few, they were able to use it to dominate and exploit the illiterate. Societies that developed political institutions, especially the modern state, were able to use this enhancement to prey on societies that lack them. The opportunities for exploitation and domination that these enhancements provided undoubtedly magnified existing inequalities.

The great historical enhancements have also led to the decline of many skills. The rise of literacy resulted in the decay of certain memory skills (and certain cultural forms, such as epic oral poetry, as well), but few people would regard that as a reason to refrain from teaching children to read and write. If there is a moral difference between biomedical and historical enhancements, it is not that the former tend to increase inequalities or opportunities for exploitation, or to result in the atrophy of skills and capacities.

It is trivially true that the historical enhancements I have listed are not *biomedical enhancements* if by the latter one means *interventions that directly improve human capabilities by the application of technologies to the human body or to human gametes or embryos*. However, to say that only biomedical enhancements (thus defined) count as the enhancement of human beings is not only arbitrary, but also smacks of a crude reductionism that identifies human beings with their biological characteristics. Nor is there any reason to think that biomedical enhancements so defined are as such any more morally problematic than enhancements of other sorts. The *means* by which we pursue enhancements may, of course, matter morally; for example, enhancements that are imposed on those who do not wish to have them would be wrong. But that is not to say that the biomedical *mode* of enhancement is in itself distinctively problematic.

To summarize: it is mistaken to assume that only biomedical enhancements deserve the title of enhancements of human beings, are irreversible, result in changes in our biology or our genetic make-up, create opportunities for injustices, or as such are especially morally problematic. What I have called the great historical enhancements share these features and they are genuine enhancements and momentous ones. Given that this is so, it is reasonable to try to place the prospect of biomedical enhancements in the historical context of human development. I shall presently argue that doing so is illuminating.

Enhancement, productivity, and well-being

Theories of economic development are misnamed: although they focus on the conditions for economic growth, they help to explain much more than the development of the economy. Such theories accord a central role to increases in productivity and to the dependence of large-scale increases in well-being on increases in productivity.[17] [*"Productivity" in the broadest sense is how good we are at using existing resources to create things we value.*]

Productivity should not be confused with various highly imperfect *proxies* for productivity, such as earning potential, or with something much narrower, namely, efficiency in the production of *economic* goods, i.e., commodities for exchange. Most academics and writers would correctly say that their computers make them more productive, better able to use the resources they have to achieve their goals; yet most would sincerely deny that their sole or even primary goal is to produce marketable goods. They rightly value their computers as cognitive enhancements that increase their ability to realize their intellectual goals and therefore as contributors to their well-being, whether or not they increase their economic productivity.

[Increased productivity does not guarantee increased well-being, because sometimes what we value turns out not to be good for us.] (For example, the increased productivity that firearms technology brought to hunting is presumably outweighed by the human destruction it enabled.) It is more accurate to say that increases in productivity often create the potential for increases in well-being that are not likely to be possible without it, while acknowledging that whether that potential is realized depends upon a number of factors.

Historically, increased productivity has been a precondition of major gains in human well-being. Increases in productivity have generally resulted from the development of technologies (such as agriculture) and institutions (including the market and the state) that are properly regarded as enhancements, as the augmentation of human capabilities.

So, the empirical link between the enhancement of human capabilities and increases in well-being is strong.

The ways in which economic development contributes to well-being are manifold: in economically developed societies there is less serious mental illness, less disease, less premature death, less disability, and less violence toward and discrimination against women, and more opportunity for people to develop their talents and pursue their own conception of the good life.

Given the link between increases in productivity and increases in well-being, it behooves us to ask whether future enhancements are likely to increase productivity and hence provide the potential for large-scale increases in well-being. Remarkably, the mainstream debate on enhancement has not asked that question.[18] The productivity-increasing effects of enhancements have been neglected.

What sorts of future biomedical enhancements might significantly increase productivity and thereby create the potential for large-scale increases in human well-being? As a first cut, the following sorts of enhancements seem most likely to fill the bill: (1) enhancements of the present cognitive capabilities of human beings (for example, increases in attention, alertness, the speed with which information is processed by the human brain, and improvements in memory), (2) enhancements that extend the duration of our lives, (3) enhancements that compress morbidity and disability near the end of life, and (4) enhancements of the human immune system. A reason for thinking that these enhancements will produce increases in productivity is that similar enhancements have done so in the past.

The potential of cognitive enhancements for increasing productivity is straightforward: other things being equal, with enhanced cognitive abilities we will be able to do what we now do more quickly and efficiently, and we also may be able to do some new things we will value. Just as adequate nutrition now allows people to function better cognitively than our malnourished ancestors did (and than malnourished people in less developed countries do now), so the right combination of diet, drugs, vitamins, and perhaps even engineered tissue or cybernetic implants may improve cognitive functioning still further. To the extent that we rightly value the things that cognitive enhancements allow us to do, cognitive enhancements will increase our well-being.

We currently lack direct evidence of the scale of increased productivity that cognitive biomedical enhancements might bring, because they are not yet widely used and their "backdoor" use through "off-label" prescription of drugs developed for the treatment of disease makes it hard to determine how widespread their use is.[19] We can, however, argue from analogy with older cognitive enhancements. For example, there is substantial evidence that in the US the use of computers has had a significant positive impact on productivity. On some estimates, information technology adds several hundred billion dollars to the monetary value of production in the US every year.[20] Gains in productivity make possible not only lower prices and hence greater access to goods and services by the less well-off, but also a larger social surplus that can be used to support the needy and mitigate the effects of natural disasters or economic downturns.

Perhaps the single most important way in which cognitive developments increase human well-being is by expanding our capacity for social coordination. Computer networks, including the World Wide Web, have greatly augmented our ability to coordinate. To a remarkable extent, these cognitive enhancements have broken or at least seriously weakened the near-monopoly that government has enjoyed as the most effective coordinating institution.

One current limitation on the effectiveness of computer technologies is the nature of the computer/human interface: what we can get out of computers depends significantly on our own limited perceptual and biological cognitive powers and our manual dexterity in using keyboards. Up until now, we have only had the option of developing new software programs—web browsers, data-mining programs, etc.—to help us get the most out of the staggering power of digital information systems. In the future, one important avenue for further cognitive enhancement and for gains in the ability to coordinate activities may well be the use of biomedical technologies to create more efficient interfacing between the brain and increasingly sophisticated computers.

Increased productivity, broadly described, requires cooperation. But collective action problems can thwart cooperation. There is evidence that more intelligent individuals are better at achieving cooperation in situations subject to the Prisoner's Dilemma, perhaps the most ubiquitous barrier to cooperation.[21] It is possible, therefore, that cognitive enhancements could facilitate cooperation and hence increase productivity, by helping to overcome such collective action problems.

If large numbers of people achieve significant cognitive enhancements, scientific progress may accelerate and this in turn may facilitate solutions to pressing problems, from the personal and social harms of a swelling elderly population, to global warming. But some relatively meager cognitive enhancements, especially in the area of memory, may yield significant benefits as well. Anders Sandberg provides two valuable illustrations.[22] First, he notes that improving the IQs of those at the lower end of the normal distribution of IQ could have a large positive impact on well-being, given that lower IQ is associated with a number of serious risks, including poverty, criminal behavior, and drug addiction. Second, Sandberg cites some rather surprising data to indicate the costs of faulty memory: lost keys result in the loss of £500 million per year in the UK.

The relationship between increased lifespan and the compression of morbidity and disability, on the one hand, and increased productivity, on the other, is straightforward. At present a 1-year increase in life expectancy increases labor productivity by 4 percent.[23] People who live to ninety and are close to the peak of their abilities until very near the end have greater capacity for being productive, other things being equal, than most people do now. They have more time to do what they value and are able to do it well for longer. This is another important way in which enhancements could increase well-being.

Whether we define "enhancement" as something that improves the "normal" abilities of humans or as an improvement on what most humans have hitherto been able to do, vaccination is an enhancement. But even if vaccination is properly described as the stimulation of the normal immune response rather than an enhancement of the normal immune system, it is nonetheless an improvement in the capability for combating diseases that human beings normally have. This enhancement has already produced significant gains in productivity, even when productivity is measured only in narrow economic terms, in addition to improving well-being in more direct ways, by lessening the burden of disease.[24]

At present our most effective tool for enhancing the human immune response is vaccination. In the future, other modes of enhancing the immune response may be possible; for example, through gene insertion, either in somatic tissue or embryos. Such alterations may qualify as enhancements not just of the immune response but of the immune system itself. Yet it would be very implausible to say that this would make them more morally problematic than vaccination.

Network effects

Literacy, numeracy, and computers are all productivity-increasing enhancements that are characterized by network effects: the value of these enhancements to the individual increases as more individuals have them. Where network effects are present, there is an obvious sense in which enhancement is *not* zero-sum: because the value of an enhancement to the individual increases as others obtain it, each individual has an interest in others getting it. In zero-sum situations, each individual has an interest in others not getting the good in question, because what others get diminishes her share of the good. Much of the literature objecting to enhancement focuses on enhancements that are "positional goods" or that would in some other way give those who have them a competitive edge.

The standard example of a positional good is being tall. It takes little capacity for inference to conclude that widespread enhancements of this sort would be futile if they were uniform. (If everybody's height increases by X percent, the tall are still tall, that is, taller than most.) It is also clear enough that in the right sort of competitive setting (e.g., a basketball game) some being taller than others benefits the former and disadvantages the latter. But it is misleading to concentrate exclusively on the ways in which enhancements may function as positional goods or create competitive advantages, while overlooking the fact that some of the most-discussed enhancements, including cognitive enhancements, are likely to have network effects. Large numbers of individuals with increased cognitive capabilities will be able to accomplish what a single individual could not, just as one can do much more with a personal computer in a world of many computer users.[25]

Network effects are one departure from the zero-sum paradigm that has tended to dominate discussions about enhancement, but there are others as well. Enhanced immunity is a good example. If others are immunized, you benefit even if you aren't, because your risk of being exposed to the infection is reduced—this is the phenomenon of herd immunity. Interventions that would bolster the normal immune system itself would also exhibit the herd immunity phenomenon.

Herd immunity is only one example of an enhancement that produces a positive externality. Generally speaking, increases in productivity are characterized by positive externalities; they tend to benefit not only the producer but others as well, at least where there are opportunities for reasonably efficient exchange. Increased productivity can enable poor people to obtain goods and services they would otherwise never have been able to afford.

Depending upon the social context, A's having an enhancement when B doesn't may give A an advantage in some zero-sum interaction that may occur between A and B (e.g., competition for a job), but it is myopic to consider this possibility alone, without considering the ways in which A's and B's interests may be not only compatible, but congruent. We should recognize that enhancements that increase productivity carry the potential for positive-sum effects, and we should take this into account in deciding whether to pursue them.

None of this is to say that all enhancements will increase productivity, be characterized by network effects or positive externalities, create opportunities for reductions in the costs of valuable goods and services, or facilitate cooperation. Some enhancements might function largely as pure positional goods, some may be mere vanities, and some may produce harms that outweigh their positive externalities. The point is that a balanced consideration of the pros and cons of enhancement should take seriously the fact that some of the most-discussed kinds of enhancements will create the potential for increases in the well-being of very large numbers of people.

Rejecting the two framing assumptions

We can now see why the first framing assumption is false and how it distorts the debate about enhancement. The Personal Goods Assumption asserts that the chief benefits of enhancements will accrue to the enhanced or their parents (whereas the risks will accrue to society as a whole, as well as to individuals). It omits consideration of the social benefits of those enhancements that will increase productivity and will be characterized by network effects or other departures from the zero-sum paradigm. Once we reject this first framing assumption, the risk–benefit picture looks quite different: we have to take seriously the social costs of *forgoing* enhancements.

The second false framing assumption is based on the first and falls with it. The Market Goods Assumption holds that (at least in liberal societies) the ill-repute of eugenics makes it highly likely that enhancements will be a private sector affair. But for enhancements that have productivity-increasing effects, this is not likely to be the case. The State may well take an interest in these enhancements and may even claim the right and indeed the obligation to foster them. Where network effect *thresholds* are present, that is, where the network effects occur only after a large number of individuals have the enhancement, the State may see its role as that of priming the pump, by providing subsidies, tax credits, or other incentives to encourage people to have the enhancement.

It is crucial to understand that the justification the State would offer for these policies would not require the illiberal assumption that the State is to create perfect human beings. Instead, it would appeal to the familiar and widely accepted idea that the State has a legitimate interest in fostering economic prosperity and increasing welfare. The justification offered would be indistinguishable from that which is used to justify education, immunization, and basic health care.

The argument thus far can now be summarized. Taken together, the first and second framing assumptions distort the debate about enhancement in two ways. First, they stack the deck against enhancement by overlooking potential major social benefits of enhancement (and potential major social costs of forgoing them). Second, they divert attention from a problem that should have a prominent place in the discussion: the possibility of State action for the development and diffusion of enhancement technologies. Focusing exclusively on the ethical problems of a private market in enhancements may blind us to even more serious perils.

Reframing the issues of distributive justice

One final feature of the rejection of the two false framing assumptions is worth pointing out. The likelihood that the State will take an interest in those enhancements that increase productivity is two-edged. On the one hand, it means that we cannot avoid thinking about the role of the State and restrict our ethical deliberations to the problems associated with a market for enhancements. On the other hand, if the State treats productivity-increasing enhancements the way it does other contributors to productivity such as basic education, immunization, and health care, then state action may actually impose *some limits on inequalities* in the distribution of these enhancements by ensuring that all have access to some "basic" level of them. If a particular enhancement had very strong productivity-enhancing effects, the failure of the State to ensure that no one lacks access to it might be as culpable as its failure to ensure that all citizens are literate or have access to immunization.

If we stick to the two false framing assumptions, we get one picture of the implications of enhancement for distributive justice and the role of the State. Taken together, the two false framing assumptions imply that the proper role of the State, from the standpoint of distributive justice, is only to constrain inequalities in the distribution of enhancements *so that the enhanced will not have an unfair competitive advantage over the unenhanced.* Focusing on the productivity-increasing dimension of the most-discussed enhancements gives a more complete picture, by recognizing an additional and perhaps more important role for the State, that of helping to ensure *that every citizen has the capacity to be an effective participant in social cooperation.*

Again, the analogy with State support for education is illuminating. From the standpoint of justice, the chief argument for the State helping to ensure that all have access to basic education is *not* that this will prevent a situation in which the educated have an unfair advantage in competitions with the uneducated. (That could be achieved by depriving *everyone* of an education.) Rather, it is that the State ought to ensure that all citizens have the productive assets needed to be able to function effectively in the predominant forms of social cooperation in their society. Similarly, once we drop the two false framing assumptions and take seriously the idea that some enhancements will significantly increase productivity, there is a case for State action to achieve a more equal distribution of those enhancements from the standpoint of what I have elsewhere called the morality of inclusion.

I am not endorsing such a role for the State. State action of this kind could be morally unacceptable or imprudent for a number of reasons. For example, the State might encourage the mass use of a memory-enhancing drug by allowing it to be sold without a prescription and it might later turn out that the drug damages other aspects of cognition or causes psychiatric disorders.[26] I simply want to indicate how changing the framing assumptions of the debate about enhancement transforms our thinking about issues of distributive justice.

Enhancement and the ethics of development

Given the potential of some future enhancements for increasing productivity and hence for creating the potential for increases in well-being, and given that the link between productivity and increased well-being has been a central feature of human development thus far, it makes sense to resituate the debate about enhancement in the larger context of the ethics of development. The ethics of development, as I understand it, is the subject matter of normative theorizing about development, undertaken in the light of the best available social science thinking about development. Here I can only indicate, in broad strokes, several ways in which thinking of the ethics of enhancement as one dimension of the ethics of development may prove illuminating.[27]

First, social science theories of so-called economic development focus not just on the effects of increases in productivity, but also on how technologies that increase productivity emerge and spread. It may turn out that theories of technological innovation and diffusion advanced by development economists will provide valuable insights into the emergence of those enhancements that increase productivity. Knowing how enhancement technologies emerge and spread will be crucial for devising effective strategies for controlling them or for fostering them.

Second, thinking of future biomedical enhancements as the latest in a series of enhancements that have played a crucial role in development may enrich the discussion of the implications of biomedical enhancements for distributive justice. I have already indicated one way in which this can occur: for enhancements that promise significant increases in productivity, the state may take an interest—and perhaps in some cases should take an interest—in ensuring that all have access to them, at least at some "basic" level of provision, as with education. More generally, thinking of the ethics of enhancement through the lens of development can encourage a greater appreciation for the complexity of the issues of distributive justice that enhancement raises. For example, it is often said that access to new enhancement technologies according to ability to pay will reinforce and perhaps even exacerbate existing inequalities or that those who have enhancements while others do not will be in a position to exploit the unenhanced. Thinking of enhancement in terms of the ethics of development may help us to understand which enhancements are of the most concern from the standpoint of distributive justice. If there is something approximating a "right to development" at the level of societies or a right of individuals to be included as an effective participant in the global basic structure, then lack of access to enhancements that significantly affect productivity may be much more serious, morally speaking, than lack of access to other enhancements.

In addition, thinking of enhancements under the rubric of development makes clear how inadequate it is to say that unless everyone has a particular enhancement, no one should, or to blithely assume that eventually everybody will catch up, due to some providential trickle-down process. Few of us would say that India should not be allowed to continue its gains in development until Ethiopia catches up; but no one acquainted with the best work in development theory would assume that disparities in development will disappear as less-developed countries benefit from some automatic trickle-down process. Social scientific thinking about development may provide crucial guidance for how to mitigate the effects of an "enhancement gap" or to shorten its duration. Work on the moral issues of development may help us to understand when such gaps are morally acceptable and when they are not.

Third, understanding enhancements within the context of development would also help us avoid the mistake of underestimating how difficult it may be to refrain from developing certain enhancements— and how hard it will be to prevent their diffusion once they are developed. For enhancements that promise significant gains in productivity, telling people they should pull up their moral socks and eschew them may prove about as effective as telling people to just say "No" to globalization.

Finally, a plausible ethics of development focuses attention squarely on three issues that economic approaches to development have only quite recently begun to take seriously but which theorists of the ethics of development have long emphasized. (1) *Under what conditions* does the adoption of various productivity-increasing technologies *actually* result in significant increases in well-being (as opposed to merely creating one necessary condition for such increases)? (2) Because increases in *aggregate* well-being are compatible with extreme inequities, aggregate measures of development are inadequate. What sorts of quantitative measures should be employed to gauge the impact on well-being of enhancements that are likely to increase productivity? (3) The character of the processes by which technologies emerge and spread can impose constraints on the possibilities for redistribution or compensation *ex post*. In particular, the character of the process may reinforce power asymmetries that prevent redistribution or compensation from being serious political options. It is therefore naïve to say that we should foster policies that "maximize innovation" and then leave it to the political process to take care of redistribution or compensation to the losers.[28] To summarize: the ethics of development approach to enhancement not only breaks the spell of the two false framing assumptions by bringing the productivity-increasing effects of enhancement into view, it also helps us avoid the naiveté and lack of ethical sensitivity that has often afflicted a purely economic approach to increasing productivity.

In Chapter Eight, I pursue the suggestion to view biomedical enhancement through the lens of the ethics of development. One of the central problems of the ethics of development is the risk of injustices posed by the incomplete or slow diffusion of beneficial innovations. The problem is that existing intellectual property rules can hinder the diffusion of beneficial technologies. Slow diffusion can not only prevent gains in well-being for the worst off, but also make them vulnerable to domination and exploitation. Biomedical enhancements are only one type of innovation among many that are subject to this problem. Technology gaps have played a role in massive injustices in the past—think, for example of their role in the evils of colonialism—and there is no reason to assume they will not do so in the future. In Chapter Nine, I propose an institutional innovation that would ameliorate the problem of incomplete or slow diffusion.

The Conservative argument

So far, I have been attempting to correct for key framing assumptions that I believe have distorted the debate. Among other things, this has involved contextualizing biomedical enhancements as just the latest instance of a major theme in human history and showing that it is a mistake to think of biomedical enhancements as being zero-sum or as only producing benefits for those who possess them. I now want to consider an objection to the approach I have been advocating:

It's true that enhancement is not new and that what we call economic development is the history of human enhancement. It's also true that some enhancements—particularly those that are likely to attract social investment—will increase productivity and that increased productivity creates the potential for increased well-being. It was a good thing that writing, numeracy, agriculture, immunization, computers, etc. were developed. But it doesn't follow that we should encourage biomedical enhancements, even if they would increase productivity and create the potential for increases in well-being. The problem is that biomedical enhancements, especially those that involve genetic changes, carry extraordinary risks, and given how well off we already are (thanks in part to past enhancements) those risks are not worth taking. So even if it would have been wrong—indeed stupid—to have forgone the major historical enhancements (if we could have), we should draw the line now.

Call this the Simple Conservative Argument.

As an argument for the conclusion that we should forgo biomedical enhancements altogether, the Simple Conservative Argument fails, for several reasons. The most obvious is that if it is supposed to provide guidance for what we should do, it is unrealistic. For reasons already noted, at least for enhancements that promise significant gains in productivity, it is unlikely that we will just say "No." Given that this is so, we should focus on how to control the pursuit of such enhancements in an ethically responsible way. I want to emphasize, however, two other objections to the Simple Conservative Argument.

First, the argument's assumption that biomedical enhancements carry uniquely high risk is dubious. It is implausible to say that the sorts of biomedical enhancements widely discussed in the enhancement debate carry significantly greater risks than enhancements we have already achieved. To take only two examples, the science that enhances so many of our capabilities has created the risk of the extinction of human life or at least of civilization by a nuclear holocaust, and the enhancement of our capability for mobility through modern transportation technologies has created the possibility of global pandemics.

Second, the Simple Conservative Argument simply *assumes* that we are now at a point at which further biomedical enhancements (or, on a more restricted version of the argument, gene-changing enhancements) will not be needed, either (1) to sustain the gains in well-being that many humans have achieved or (2) to make these gains available to those who now lack them. But this assumption is also highly dubious. We may need further enhancements, perhaps even gene-changing enhancements, either to ensure that we in the developed countries continue to enjoy the benefits of past enhancements or to help close the gap between us and the people of less-developed countries, or for both reasons.

Here are some examples of enhancements that might be needed either for holding our own or for providing the benefits of previous enhancements to all.

1. Enhancement of existing capacities for impulse control, sympathy, altruism, or moral imagination, through pharmaceutical or genetic interventions. Given the current human propensity for violence, the prevalence of ideologies that fuel it, and the availability of highly destructive weapons technologies to individuals and small groups not subject to effective political control, we might come to need such interventions as part of a more complex strategy for catastrophic violence.[29]

2. Enhancement of the human capacity for extracting nutrients from current foods and perhaps even the development of the ability to extract nutrients from items that humans have never consumed before.[30] Such enhancements might be extremely valuable if global warming or massive environmental damage due to the accumulation of toxins significantly reduce the capacity to produce standard food crops.

3. Enhancement of the "normal" viability of human gametes and/or embryos, or the invention of new reproductive technologies, in order to counteract a decrease in fertility, an increase in lethal mutations, or a rise in the rate of cancers due to environmental toxins.

4. Enhancements to help us to adapt physiologically to climate change. (For example, drugs or gene therapies to improve the body's capacity for thermal regulation or the skin's resistance to cancers.)

5. Enhancements of the immune system and/or enhancements of the body's ability to repair damaged tissues in order to compress morbidity in countries in which life-expectancy has already increased significantly, so as to avoid the breakdown of social welfare systems under the strain of a large population of chronically ill elderly people.

6. Enhancements of the immune system to accelerate the development of resistance to virulent emerging infectious diseases in an era of globalization.

This rebuttal of the Simple Conservative Argument is just that; it is *not* an argument in favor of enhancements across the board or even an argument for a presumption in favor of pursuing biomedical enhancements. It is a critique of the smug assumptions that lie behind the recommendation to put the brakes on human enhancement generally or to eschew biomedical or genetic enhancements in particular. The Simple Conservative Argument may have considerable bite when applied to some particular proposal for enhancement, by prompting us to consider whether the enhancement in question carries a significant risk of undermining something we already have and value and whether, if it does, the enhancement would be worth the risk. But the Conservative Argument cannot enable us to draw a bright line between the historical enhancements and biomedical enhancements, and thus cannot undermine my proposal for exploring the ethics of enhancement through the lens of the ethics of development.

There are other Conservative arguments. The Simple Conservative Argument is only the most obvious. Chapter Five is devoted to a more thorough exploration of the relationship between the best Conservative moral–political thought and enhancement. My criticism of the Simple Conservative Argument in the present chapter has a limited aim: to show that it is a fundamental mistake to assume that enhancements are valuable only for the purpose of achieving *improvements* in well-being. In some cases, improvements of particular normal human capacities may be needed to prevent things from getting worse, perhaps much worse. Thus, in Chapter Five I will argue that, paradoxically, the characteristic Conservative admonition to appreciate and preserve the goods we now enjoy can *require* enhancements.

The statement that enhancements may be needed not to make things better but to keep them from getting worse is consistent with the definition of enhancement introduced in Chapter One. Enhancement as I defined it there is a local affair: it is the improvement of a capacity or function, with no assumption that this means an improvement in well-being overall, either for the individual who is enhanced or for society. So, it is quite consistent to say that an enhancement (for example, of the body's capacity to fight infectious disease or of the mind's ability to solve complex problems such as climate change) might be needed to prevent a worsening of our condition, even if it did not make us better off in a more positive sense.

A more fundamental framing issue: balancing versus exclusionary reasons

So far I have argued for three theses. (1) We should reorient thinking about the ethics of enhancement by abandoning two false framing assumptions that have distorted the debate. (2) Once we see that some enhancements will increase productivity and create the possibility of large-scale gains in well-being, the case for pursuing them becomes stronger, other things being equal. (3) It is fruitful to view the ethics of enhancement as one important dimension of the ethics of development. I have proceeded on the assumption that it makes sense to weigh the pros and cons (or, very broadly construed, the risks and benefits) of various biomedical enhancements. Call this the Balancing Approach.

This assumption can be challenged, too. It would have to be abandoned *if there are any conclusive moral reasons against biomedical enhancement that are available to us now*—prior to the exercise of trying to take all the pros and cons of this or that enhancement into account. If there are such reasons, then my whole approach has been wrong. If there are such reasons, then they are exclusionary reasons in this sense: they are so morally potent that they rule out appeals to the benefits of enhancement. Call the view that we already have conclusive reasons against biomedical enhancements the Conclusive Reasons View. According to the Conclusive Reasons View, we already have reasons against enhancement that are so powerful as to exclude any countervailing considerations, so the case against enhancement is already conclusively made.

Two ways of thinking about the ethics of enhancement

If the Conclusive Reasons View is correct, then the Balancing Approach is wrong. My argument thus far has simply assumed the truth of the Balancing Approach in this sense: I have proceeded on the assumption that there are no conclusive reasons against biomedical enhancements *ex ante*, and then explored some important reasons in favor of some biomedical enhancements that have been neglected in the debate. The Conclusive Reasons View rejects the Balancing Approach and hence calls my approach into question.

Note that the Balancing Approach does *not* assume that all the pros and cons of enhancement are commensurable, much less quantifiable. Rather, the idea is that the proper way to think about the ethics of enhancement is to try to articulate all the considerations in favor of and against enhancements of various sorts, to reflect on them in the light of our most important moral values, and then try to make an impartial, factually informed, all-things-considered judgment about what to do, or at least to try to identify a range of morally acceptable options. The Balancing Approach is a commonsensical view, because it recommends that we think about technologies that provide enhancements in the same way we think about technologies in general—namely, by recognizing that they can be used for good or for ill. It invites us to consider the pros and cons (or costs and benefits broadly construed) and then to pursue or avoid various enhancements depending upon where the balance of reasons lies.

The Balancing Approach does *not* assume consequentialism, the view that the rightness of an action depends solely on its consequences. It does not assume that all pros and cons can be aggregated on a single scale of value or that the goal is to maximize aggregate value or that there are no non-consequentialist reasons against enhancements. It merely says that it is appropriate to look both at the considerations in favor of enhancement and those against and to strive for a judgment that reflects a proper appreciation of both. It leaves open the possibility that some of the considerations against enhancement may be deontological, rather than consequentialist in nature.

I now want to suggest that some of the most vocal critics of biomedical enhancement, including Fukuyama, Kass, Sandel, and Habermas, could be understood as trying to make a case against the Balancing Approach and in favor of the Conclusive Reasons View. All of these critics proceed as if they subscribe to the Conclusive Reasons View: they lay out what they take to be powerful reasons against enhancement (or in Habermas's case a particular mode of enhancement, the genetic engineering of human embryos). They do *not* then go on to discuss considerations *in favor* of enhancement and then argue for an all things considered judgment against enhancement. They proceed as if undertaking any sort of balancing is not necessary. Indeed, their tone sometimes suggests that such an undertaking would be not only misguided, but would also betray a kind of moral obtuseness. This suggests that they endorse the Conclusive Reasons View.

In the next chapter, I examine concerns about the relationship between the pursuit of enhancement and character. In Chapter Five,

I examine the idea that enhancement is a threat to our human nature or an improper interference with the natural. In both cases, the anti-enhancement views I critically evaluate can be seen in either of two distinct ways: as efforts to provide conclusive reasons against enhancement—to show that further consideration of the pros and cons of enhancement is unnecessary and inappropriate—or as important considerations to be taken into account in a comprehensive weighing of pros and cons. Until the work of Chapters Three and Four is done, we will not be in a position to know whether there are conclusive reasons available to us at this time for rejecting biomedical enhancements across the board or for eschewing the enhancement enterprise. Thus, the most I can hope to accomplish in the present chapter is to show that there is a *prima facie* case for undertaking the enhancement enterprise. By the close of the final chapter I hope to have shown that the balance of reasons favors the enhancement enterprise, at least for now.

A provisional case for the enhancement enterprise

When we consider the potential benefits of biomedical enhancements, recognizing that they may be needed not just for improvements, but also to preserve what we have, the idea of banning biomedical enhancements altogether and only allowing biomedical technology to be used to prevent or treat disease is quickly seen to be both imprudent and morally irresponsible. When we reflect on the central role of enhancements in human history and on the fact that biomedical enhancements will inevitably continue to emerge from efforts to prevent and treat disease, we see that the idea of banning enhancements is unrealistic. Given that a ban on biomedical enhancements is both unwise and unrealistic, there are two main alternatives: "backdoor enhancement" (living in a society in which biomedical enhancement is not recognized as a legitimate endeavor in its own right, subject to institutional controls, but where biomedical enhancements emerge in an unplanned fashion from efforts to prevent and treat disease); or undertaking the enhancement enterprise, acknowledging that biomedical enhancements, like other enhancements, can be a legitimate aim of individuals and of society, and then developing an appropriate institutional framework within which it can occur.

Elements of the enhancement enterprise

The idea of a society undertaking the enhancement enterprise requires careful explication. The first thing to emphasize is that the proposal is *not* a prescription for what every society, no matter what its political institutions and political culture are like, should do. It is restricted to well-established, reasonably liberal constitutional democracies: societies in which there is democratic accountability through fair, periodic elections, separation of powers (including an independent judiciary), a system of entrenched civil and political rights that protect not only individuals but minority groups as well, and a robust civil society that includes nongovernmental organizations dedicated to protecting civil and political rights, including reproductive rights. Many societies meet these criteria, as I understand them, including most European countries, South Africa, the UK, the United States, Canada, Australia, New Zealand, Japan, South Korea, Taiwan, and a growing cohort of countries in Latin America. This list is meant to be illustrative, not exhaustive.

For it to be advisable for a country to embark on the enhancement enterprise, it must have both institutions and a political culture that make it more reasonable to try to subject the development and deployment of biomedical enhancement technologies to social control under the democratic rule of law than to refrain from doing so out of fear that the State will hijack biomedical enhancements for its own purposes, at the expense of the general population or of some disfavored minorities. In some societies, undertaking the enhancement enterprise might be riskier than "backdoor enhancement." In particular, a society that was deficient from the standpoint of constitutionally entrenched civil and political rights or was authoritarian rather than democratic might run an unacceptable risk of a new State-driven, coercive eugenics if it invested in biomedical enhancements.

What would undertaking the enhancement enterprise amount to? Several key components of the enterprise need to be distinguished. Each feature confers significant advantages over "backdoor enhancement," given the background assumption that the society in question has the liberal-democratic institutions and political culture described earlier. (1) It means recognizing that enhancement can be a legitimate aim both for individuals and for society as a whole and that there is no good reason to presume that biomedical enhancements, as a class, are especially morally problematic. One important implication of this first element of the enhancement enterprise is a clear rejection of any attempt at a ban on biomedical enhancements as such, and a public recognition that those who seek to ban particular biomedical enhancements must make their case for doing so in the public arena of the society's political processes, giving reasons that reflect a recognition that enhancement is a legitimate, long-standing, and often an admirable human activity. Another is that the pursuit of enhancements ought not to be shoehorned into the medical model. In making decisions concerning the use of biomedical enhancements, people should have access to the expert advice and skills of biomedical professionals, under appropriate conditions of informed consent, without having to convince anyone that they have a disease or disorder. (2) It means acknowledging that the development of biomedical enhancements is an institutional phenomenon—the product of the interplay of scientific institutions, government, and the market—and that guiding and controlling the creation and deployment of biomedical enhancement technologies will require institutional action and perhaps even the development of new institutions, not just individual moral resolve. (3) It means recognizing that considerations of distributive justice are an integral part of a sound institutional approach to the challenges of enhancement. In particular, as I argue in Chapter Eight, it may be necessary to build effective measures to avoid injustices in the distribution of valuable biomedical enhancement technologies into the innovation process itself (for example, by modifying intellectual property rules). (4) It means recognizing that although biomedical enhancement can be a legitimate social aim, it is only one among others and should be pursued within the constraints of reasonable priority setting. Treating biomedical enhancement as a legitimate endeavor allows informed, systematic public deliberation about the opportunity costs of biomedical enhancements vis-à-vis other social goods. (5) Undertaking the enhancement enterprise means making a serious effort to ensure that the best available information is available both for public policy decisions concerning the development and deployment of biomedical enhancement technologies, and for individual decision making concerning their use. A society that undertakes the enhancement enterprise recognizes a societal obligation to gather information on the risks and benefits of various enhancements, to monitor their long-term effects, and to reassess and if need be reverse its policy decisions in the light of this information. In contrast, if biomedical enhancement enters through the backdoor, it will be more difficult to assess its actual effects and to detect problems earlier rather than later.

It is important to avoid a misunderstanding: a society's engaging in the enhancement enterprise does not mean that that it expropriates biomedical enhancement, making it purely, or even primarily, a collective enterprise. On the contrary, a central feature of the enhancement enterprise, as I use that phrase, is to allow competent individuals, under conditions of accurate information about the likely effects of various enhancements, to make decisions about whether or not to employ them and to create favorable conditions for innovation, subject to the demands of distributive justice. In brief, the enhancement enterprise entails carving out a space for individual freedom to use or not to use enhancements, and for private enterprise to play a key role in the development of biomedical enhancement technologies.

In this chapter, I hope to have made a strong *prima facie* case for societies of a certain sort provisionally undertaking the enhancement enterprise. Whether the *prima facie* case is a convincing case all things considered depends upon whether there are countervailing reasons— considerations against biomedical enhancement that outweigh the attractions of the enhancement enterprise. In the next six chapters I articulate and critically evaluate the most prominent candidates for such countervailing reasons: concerns about the implications of biomedical enhancement for character (Chapter Three), worries about biomedical enhancements putting human nature or the natural at risk (Chapter Four), the best insights of the Conservative tradition in moral and political thought (Chapter Five), the risk of unintended bad consequences (Chapter Six) the possibility that enhancement might undermine the moral status of persons (Chapter Seven), and the risk that enhancements will worsen existing distributive injustices (Chapter Eight).

Notes

1. See Leon Kass (1997), "The Wisdom of Repugnance." *New Republic* 216 (22): 17–26.
2. Michael Sandel (2007), *The Case Against Perfection: Ethics in the Age of Genetic Engineering* (Harvard University Press) pp. 99–100.

3. See, for example, Francis Fukuyama (2002), *Our Posthuman Future* (New York: Farrar, Straus and Giroux), pp. 9–10.
4. For a discussion of potential "evolutionary harms" associated with genetic enhancement technology, see R. Powell (forthcoming), "The Evolutionary Biological Implications of Human Genetic Engineering," *Journal of Medicine and Philosophy.*
5. My focus in this essay is on what might be called the "mainstream debate" about the ethics of enhancement, namely the controversy among bioethicists that focuses squarely on the ethical issues. I do not consider the less ethically focused popular "posthumanist" or futurists literatures.
6. There are frequent comparisons between current uses of performance-enhancing drugs in sports competitions and future enhancements of cognitive and physical abilities. For an especially clear example, see Michael Sandel 2004, supra note 2, p. 52.
7. Some liberal thinkers who favor a permissive policy on the availability of biomedical enhancements, especially those that prospective parents might use to enhance the capacities of their offspring, have apparently thought it unnecessary to spell out the potential social benefits of these technologies, because they think that (a) biomedical enhancement falls under the scope of reproductive liberty (or liberty more generally) and that (b) reproductive liberty (or liberty more generally) is of such great value that the consideration of social benefits is unnecessary. I am grateful to Nicholas Agar for calling this point to my attention. My strategy is to consider the potential individual and social benefits of biomedical enhancement, as well as the costs, and to avoiding hanging the case for the enhancement project on what I consider to be a dubious view about the overwhelming value of reproductive liberty (or liberty more generally). Even though liberty is extremely important, considerations of costs, and more particularly, of serious harm, can provide good reasons to regulate or limit it.
8. Mark S. Frankel (2003), Inheritable Genetic Modification and a Brave New World. *Hastings Center Report* 33(2): 31–36; Francis Fukuyama (2002), *Our Posthuman Future* (New York: Farrar, Straus and Giroux) p. 32. Diane Paul. (2005) Genetic Engineering and Eugenics: The Uses of History. In *Is Human Nature Obsolete?* Harold W. Baillie and Timothy K. Casey (eds.) (Cambridge, MA: MIT Press) pp. 123–152.
9. In his latest valuable contribution to the literature on enhancement John Harris recognizes that enhancement is already ubiquitous in human life, but he does not explain the connection among enhancement, productivity, and well-being. See John Harris (2007), *Enhancing Evolution* (Princeton: Princeton University Press).
10. If language was a crucial feature in the differentiation of humans from other hominids with whom we share a common ancestor, then it would be misleading to say that language is a *human* enhancement, an improvement

of *human* beings; instead it would be an enhancement of pre-humans that helped make them human. In pointing out the great benefits of literacy as a cognitive enhancement, I am not assuming that the benefits are evenly distributed. As Nicholas Agar has pointed out to me, some people may suffer from learning disabilities that prevent them from reaping as much benefit from literacy as others do.

11. For one of the most valuable articles presently available on cognitive enhancement, see Anders Sandberg, "Cognitive Enhancement: Upgrading the Brain" (unpublished).

12. See Jared Diamond (1997), *Guns, Germs and Steel: The Fates of Human Societies* (W.W. Norton and Co.).

13. Robert W. Fogel (2004), *The escape from hunger and premature death, 1700–2100: Europe, America, and the Third World* (Cambridge University Press).

14. Anneliese A. Pontius (1982), Face Representation Linked with Literacy Level in Colonial American Tombstone Engravings and Third World Preliterates' Drawings. Toward a Cultural-Evolutionary Neurology. *Cellular and Molecular Sciences* 38: 577–581.

15. See S.A. Tishkoff (2007), F.A. Reed, A. Ranciaro *et al.*, "Convergent adaptation of human lactase persistence in Africans and Europeans." *Nature Genetics* 39(1): 31–40.

16. For a discussion of distributive justice issues in the context of genetic enhancement, see Allen Buchanan, Dan W. Brock, Norman Daniels, and Daniel Wikler (2001), *From Chance to Choice: Genetics and Justice*, (Cambridge University Press), Chapter 3.

17. For a prominent example, see David S. Landes (2003), *The Unbound Prometheus: Technological Change and Industrial Development in Western Europe from 1750 to the Present, 2003* (Cambridge University Press). For a fascinating analysis of the contribution of increases in productivity to the moral improvement of human beings, see Benjamin M. Freedman (2005), *The Moral Consequences of Economic Growth* (Knopf).

18. Anders Sandberg (2009), "The Economics of Cognitive Development," in *Enhancing Human Capabilities*, Julian Savulescu *et al.* (eds.) (Oxford: Wiley-Blackwell Publishers). Nick Bostrom and Rebecca Roache (2010), "Smart Policy: Cognitive Enhancement and the Public Interest," in *Enhancing Human Capacities*, Julian Savulescu *et al.* (eds.) (Oxford: Wiley Blackwell).

19. For a study on the non-medical use of prescription stimulants among US college students, see Sean Esteban McCabe, John R. Knight, Christian J. Teter, and Henry Wechsler (2005), "Non-medical use of prescription stimulants among US college students: prevalence and correlates from a national survey," *Addiction* 99: 96–106.

20. Sandberg 2009, supra note 14.
21. G. Jones (2008), "Are Smarter Groups More Cooperative? Evidence From Prisoner's Dilemma Experiments, 1959–2003," *Journal of Economic Behavior and Organization* 68(3–4): 489–497. In Prisoner's Dilemma situations, it is rational for each individual to defect from cooperation, but the result is an outcome that is suboptimal from the standpoint of all.
22. Sandberg 2009, supra note 12.
23. According to Bloom *et al.*, "This [4 percent] is a relatively large effect, indicating that increased expenditures on improving health might be justified purely on the grounds of their impact on labor productivity, quite apart from the direct effect of improved health on welfare." D.E. Bloom, D. Canning, and J. Sevilla (2004), "The effect of health on economic growth: a production function approach," *World Development* 32(1): 1–13, p. 11.
24. Vaccination has proven to be a valuable means of improving human health because of costs averted via the direct medical impact of vaccines (i.e., through prevented illnesses). Interestingly, however, recent economic studies suggest that traditional cost-effectiveness and cost–benefit analyses often ignore the broader economic impact of vaccination. For example, the Global Alliance for Vaccination and Immunization (GAVI) has a vaccine package for seventy-five low-income countries that, if implemented, could provide an economic rate of return nearly equal to primary education. See D.E. Bloom, D. Canning, and M. Weston (2005), "The Value of Vaccination," *World Economics* 6: 15–39, p. 35.
25. There is another reason why focusing exclusively or even mainly on positional goods in the enhancement debate is misguided. As Harry Brighouse and Adam Swift point out, goods can have positional and nonpositional aspects, and whether a good is positional or how deleterious its positional aspect is may be subject to social control, because both depend upon how the good is embedded in social relationships that may be amenable to modification. Harry Brighouse and Adam Swift (2006), "Equality, Priority, and Positional Goods," *Ethics* 116: 471–497.
26. I thank David Goldstein for this example.
27. Note that my claim is not that the ethics of enhancement can be reduced to or fully subsumed under the ethics of development.
28. Matthew DeCamp forcefully makes this point in his outstanding dissertation, "Global Health: A Normative Analysis of Intellectual Property Rights and Global Distributive Justice," Duke University, 2007.
29. Nick Bostrom (2004), "The Future of Human Evolution," *Death and Anti-Death: Tow Hundred Years after Kant, Fifty Years After Turing*, Charles Tandy (ed.) (Palo Alto: Ria University Press), pp. 339–371.
30. At present human beings, unlike most mammals (primates excluded) cannot biosynthesize vitamin C, due to a mutation (approximately 40 million years ago) that causes the inactivation of a gene for the production

of a critical enzyme. It may become possible to change this in the future. See Michael N. Haa, Frank L. Grahama, Chantalle K. D'Souzaa, William J. Mullera, Suleiman A. Igdouraa, and Herb E. Schellhorn (2004), "Functional rescue of vitamin C synthesis deficiency in human cells using adenoviral-based expression of murine l-gulono-γ-lactone oxidasestar," *Genomics* 83(3): 482–492.

CHAPTER THREE

Character

Sorting out character concerns

A striking feature of the enhancement literature is the prominence of concerns about character. Character concerns are voiced by thinkers across the political spectrum. Not only conservatives, but also many who take liberal stances on most issues, are deeply worried about the implications of enhancement for character. "Character" here means moral character; so concerns about character can be framed in terms of the language of virtue and vice. They can also be framed in terms of values.

Expressivist versus consequentialist concerns

Two kinds of character concerns need to be distinguished: expressivist and consequentialist. The expressivist (or *non*consequentialist) concern is that the pursuit of enhancements, independently of its consequences, itself *indicates* bad character. Consequentialist concerns are predictions that the pursuit of enhancements will *result* in a worsening of our characters.

· seems possible

The strongest version of the expressivist concern is the thesis that a stable desire to enhance (rather than merely to treat or prevent diseases) is itself a manifestation of vice (or at least of a deficiency of virtue). A weaker version is the thesis that the desire to enhance is usually or predominantly the expression of a vice (or a deficiency of virtue). The stronger version is strong indeed: it implies that the voluntary pursuit of enhancements *always* has morally tainted motivational roots and that the roots extend deep into the person, forming part of her character.

The weaker version avoids this extraordinary claim, but is nonetheless committed to the ambitious empirical generalization that the pursuit of enhancement usually (or at least very often) is an expression of bad character. The stronger version claims that a stable desire for enhancement, or we might also say, a commitment to enhancement, *in itself* is conclusive evidence of deficiency of character. The weaker version asserts that the pursuit of enhancement is *likely to be* the expression of vice or distorted values and is therefore substantial *evidence* of bad character. A frustrating aspect of the debate is that those who voice character concerns do not make it clear whether they are making the stronger or the weaker claim.

Before attempting to make sense of expressivist character concerns, I want to point out that there are two reasons to be wary of any attempt to dissociate entirely the expressive dimension from consequences. First, as Aristotle noted, repeated bad actions can result in bad character, just as repeated good actions can result in good character. In other words, a pattern of actions of the sort that are typical expressions of bad character can *result* in bad character. Second, according to mainstream virtue ethics theory, having the virtues is conducive to or constitutive of, personal well-being: a virtuous individual, at least if he lives under reasonably favorable conditions, tends to flourish. Nevertheless, the claim that the commitment to or stable desire for enhancement either is in itself a defect of character or is substantial evidence of such a defect is interesting and worth probing, independently of further concerns about the consequences of the pursuit of enhancement for character.

My strategy will be to sort out, spell out, and evaluate a cluster of concerns about biomedical enhancement that are presented as concerns about character, with special emphasis on those of the expressivist variety. I will also attempt to discern when the concern is really expressivist and when it is consequentialist. In the end I will argue that the most extreme expressivist concerns are ill-founded, that often what appear to be expressivist concerns turn out to be consequentialist concerns, and that if consequentialist concerns are to constitute strong arguments against enhancement much more will have to be done to provide empirical support for the very strong and sweeping empirical claims on which they rely.

Character concerns or objections?

So far I have spoken of character *concerns*, not objections or arguments to anti-enhancement conclusions. That is because worries about character exhibit one of the frustrating features of the enhancement debate I flagged in Chapter One: it is hard to know what the practical implications of various critiques of enhancement are because it is not clear exactly what the critics are saying. This may be especially true in the case of character concerns.

To help clarify, it is useful to distinguish between objections and concerns as follows: an *objection* to enhancement is an argument for the conclusion that enhancement across the board or certain enhancements or types of enhancements (or certain types, in certain circumstances) are undesirable. One could also construe some concerns about enhancement as arguments for the conclusion that the enhancement enterprise (as I defined it in Chapter Two) ought not to be undertaken. A *concern* about enhancement is merely a consideration that counts against enhancement, either across the board or against certain enhancements or types of enhancements (in certain circumstances, etc). All objections are concerns, but not all concerns are objections. Concerns, as such, are merely "cons"; objections are conclusory. In other words, concerns may not add up to an anti-enhancement conclusion. Here are the main alternatives worth considering.

1. Expressivist character concerns are objections to pursuing any bio-medical enhancements whatsoever (i.e., they constitute arguments for the anti-enhancement view, the conclusion that we should reject biomedical enhancements across the board).

2. Expressivist character concerns are objections to pursuing some particular biomedical enhancements (under certain conditions).

3. Expressivist character concerns are objections to pursuing the enhancement enterprise—i.e., the conclusion that is supposed to follow from them is that a reasonably liberal, democratic society ought not to legitimate and support the pursuit of biomedical enhancements.

4. Expressivist character concerns are (merely) considerations to be taken into account by individuals in deciding whether to pursue enhancements and by society, through its political processes, in deciding whether to undertake the enhancement enterprise—i.e., they should be weighed against the reasons in favor of enhancement.

If character concerns are understood as in (1) they can be quickly dismissed for two reasons. First, even if it were true that the pursuit of enhancement is *always* driven solely by bad character, it would not follow from this that enhancement is morally impermissible. That is a confusion, because one can perform the right act as a result of bad motivation. If the benefits of an enhancement were great enough—especially, if they were morally admirable—and if they were achieved through morally acceptable means, then the fact that their achievement was motivationally tainted might not be a sufficient reason to forgo them. Consider an analogy: suppose it were true that people or, perhaps somewhat more plausibly, nations, only cooperate for selfish reasons; if the benefits of cooperation are great enough, cooperation may be not only morally permissible but also morally obligatory, in spite of the seedy character of the motivation that makes it possible.

Second, and more importantly, as I have already noted, it is *not* true that the pursuit of enhancement is always the expression of bad motives or defective character. Those who voice character concerns have given us no good reason to disregard the commonsensical assumption that the pursuit of enhancement can be and in fact is sometimes driven by morally respectable motives and need not betray bad character or distorted values. To take only one example from many in Chapter One: a person may pursue cognitive enhancements—whether in the form of computers or drugs—not because she wants to get ahead in competitions with others, but because she wants to accomplish some worthy goals for which greater cognitive functioning is needed, or simply because she enjoys pursuits that are more cognitively demanding, independently of the results they produce. For example, a scientist might seek a better software program for gene sequencing in order to have a better chance of finding a cure for some horrible genetic disease. Saying that what people "really" want when they pursue enhancements is mastery[1] is about as plausible as saying that all people "really" want is pleasure or that all they "really" do is pursue their self-interest. Human motivation is a bit more complex and variegated than that. Making uncharitable and unfounded assumptions about the motives of someone one disagrees with is a very old (and very sleazy) rhetorical trick.

On interpretation (2), the character concern is supposed to provide an objection, not to enhancement across the board, but to certain enhancements or certain enhancements under certain conditions. The difficulty

[handwritten margin notes:]
interesting concept to follow up on
ties into thoughts of selfish incentives in IMA
this is my current view actually

here is that the claims made by those who voice character concerns seem to be too general to allow such discrimination. For example, Sandel, as we have already seen, seems to think that the pursuit of enhancement *as such* betrays an unseemly craving for mastery or perfection.[2] But if that were so, then it is hard to see how he can avoid a condemnation of enhancement—and not just biomedical enhancement—across the board. This means he would be committed to condemning education, science, literacy, computers, and every technology that extends human capacities.[3]

Truth

Later, I will explore in considerable detail the idea that under certain conditions the pursuit of enhancement can betray bad character or distorted values; but, unlike those who voice character concerns, I will try to say something informative about what those conditions are. For now I will only observe that if character concerns are understood according to interpretation (2), they are of little interest unless a lot more can be said—and plausibly said—about when the pursuit of enhancement does and when it does not betray bad character.

If character concerns are understood according to interpretation (3), the result is not promising for the critics of enhancement, for reasons already indicated. Whether the enhancement enterprise is a good idea depends in the first instance on whether the expected benefits are great enough, given the costs, and on whether those benefits can be achieved through morally permissible means. It also depends upon whether we are better off making issues concerning the development and use of enhancements a legitimate topic for democratic deliberation, rather than allowing enhancements to come through the backdoor, unscrutinized and unregulated, as spin-offs from treatments.

important

Notice that I am using "costs" and "benefits" here in a very broad sense, so that negative effects on character are included. But recall that at this point we are not considering the *effects* of the pursuit of enhancements on character; we are considering expressivist concerns. What would have to be true about the connection between character and the enhancement enterprise for expressivist concerns about character to provide a plausible argument for the conclusion that we should not pursue the enhancement enterprise?

Perhaps the idea is this: the motivational roots of the pursuit of enhancement are so likely to be seriously tainted that we should forgo the enhancement project in order to close the door to the opportunity to express bad character. On this line of thinking, the chief concern is nonconsequentialist in this sense: the problem is not that pursuing the enhancement enterprise will cause our character to deteriorate further (though that might also happen), but that it will provide a spacious arena in which our already deficient character will be given free play. If we care about character, we should avoid situations in which our vices will be given even greater scope for rearing their ugly heads.

Is this interpretation of the expressivist character concern cogent? Should we forgo all the benefits that the enhancement enterprise is likely to bring in order to prevent ourselves from having whatever new opportunities for exhibiting the character defects the enhancement enterprise is likely to create? The answer to that question depends on four factors: (1) how bad our character defects are now, (2) how much additional scope for exhibiting them the enhancement enterprise would provide, (3) how bad the risk of this greater scope for vice is compared to the benefits of the enhancement enterprise, and (4) whether we are able to employ effective and morally permissible strategies to prevent ourselves from acting viciously when confronted with the new opportunities for doing so that the enhancement enterprise will present. But it also depends on something else: whether the enhancement enterprise is likely to produce *improvements in our character*.

Here we are confronted with a heavy irony. Some of the most vocal critics of enhancement claim that those who regard enhancement more favorably fail to take character concerns seriously enough. On interpretation (3), they also claim that the social legitimation of enhancement—embarking on the enhancement enterprise—will give such great scope for vice that we ought to avoid it. But in making this latter claim they assume a rather pessimistic view *about human character*: to them, our embarking on the enhancement enterprise is like a group of alcoholics pooling their resources to open more bars. Such pessimism raises an obvious question: If we are so vicious that we must avoid giving any further scope for the exercise of our vices, shouldn't we be doing what we reasonably can to become less vicious? Those who invoke character concerns overlook the possibility that some enhancements could improve our character.[4]

Their assessment of the risks to character that enhancement poses presents human character as fragile and too puny to resist the temptations that enhancement technologies will bring. Given this rather unflattering view of our character, it appears to be a good candidate for enhancement. Instead of arguing that enhancement is too risky to our character, why not proceed in the opposite direction and argue that, given how deficient our character is, we may need moral enhancement technologies? Especially if we acknowledge that our character is constrained—perhaps even seriously impaired—by our evolved biology, we ought to consider the possibility of biomedically enhancing it. After all, what biological evolution reliably produces (and then only approximately and fleetingly) is reproductively fit organisms. Moreover, the dominant view among evolutionary psychologists is that the basic features of human motivation were shaped in the Pleistocene era, to help us function in the face of radically different environmental challenges from those we now face. There is no reason to assume that evolution has produced human beings whose character is adequate to the demands of morality, much less the demands of morality in our current situation. Nor is there any reason to assume that the limitations that biological evolution places on human character can be fully overcome by culture. Perhaps human culture has produced new moral challenges that we are incapable of meeting, without the help of biomedical enhancements.[5]

How would moral enhancement by biomedical means work? There are two main possibilities, both admittedly quite speculative—though less speculative than the claim that *whatever* the benefits of enhancement turn out to be, they will be outweighed by the additional scope for vice that the enhancement project would create. On the one hand, certain cognitive enhancements could help us be more virtuous, to the extent that virtuous behavior depends on our cognitive powers. Virtues involve sound judgments and sound judgments depend in part on good information processing and reasoning.[6] In addition, there is considerable evidence that normal human memory is extremely fallible. To the extent that we are committed to the virtues of veracity and to avoiding the vice of self-deception and the moral errors it fosters, we should be deeply concerned about the often self-serving character of our flawed memory. Biomedical enhancements of memory might, therefore, make us more virtuous. Finally, psychologists have shown that human beings are prone to certain cognitive biases, and some of these biases can contribute to the patterns of bad behavior that were traditionally called vices.[7] If cognitive enhancements reduced these biases, this, too, would facilitate moral

checks out so far (margin note)

improvement. For all of these reasons and more, there is reason to believe that some cognitive enhancements could help improve character.

Alternatively, enhancements of the moral emotions could also make us less vicious or more virtuous. For example, it may become possible to increase our capacity for sympathy or for moral imagination—for vividly entertaining possibilities other than the status quo, for fully appreciating the impact of our actions on others. Notice that these possibilities do *not* presuppose genetic determinism: they depend only on the reasonable assumption that biotechnologies could contribute to our achieving better character, not on the assumption that having good character is determined solely or even predominantly by biological factors.

There is a further irony. Some critics of enhancement hold *both* that human beings are so prone to vice that we cannot afford to create the temptations that the enhancement enterprise would bring *and* that human beings as they now exist are so morally admirable that we should avoid anything, including the enhancement enterprise, that might destroy or damage our "humanity." In Chapter Six, I will argue that how much risk we should tolerate in efforts to enhance ourselves depends in part on how flawed we are, and that evolutionary biology reinforces two commonsense beliefs: first, that human beings have serious defects, and, second, that some of our defects impose substantial limitations on character. If it turns out that a view of human nature that is informed by evolutionary biology provides a rather pessimistic picture of human character, and if biomedical technologies can ameliorate some of these defects, then *taking character seriously may speak in favor of rather than against the enhancement enterprise.* In Chapter Five, when I explore relationships between conservative thought and the enhancement debate, I carefully explore this possibility.

On each of the first three interpretations above, then, character concerns do not look cogent. The fourth interpretation, according to which character concerns are "cons" to be weighed against the "pros" of enhancements, on a case-by-case basis, makes them more plausible. There are several serious risks that could be lumped together under the heading "character concerns" that a judicious consideration of the enhancement enterprise ought to take into account. They fall into four groupings: (1) concerns about perfectionism and the quest for mastery; (2) concerns about gratitude, or, more accurately, about due appreciation of existing goods; (3) concerns about self-manipulation or

First reason B. MD, E that really is appealing to me (margin note)

Rmmbr (margin note)

true that these are incompatible p. DoV. (margin note)

objectification; and (4) concerns about inauthenticity. I will argue that even when taken together, these valid character concerns do not provide conclusive reasons—at present—to oppose the enhancement enterprise. Instead, their proper role is that of input into the complex task of determining *how* to pursue it.

Enhancement, perfectionism, and the quest for mastery

Perhaps the most widely discussed character concern comes from Michael Sandel. For him, the very effort to enhance human beings expresses morally flawed attitudes, values, and character defects. As we saw in Chapter One, Sandel claims that those who pursue enhancement evidence a boundless craving for mastery and for perfection and thereby exhibit a lack of proper appreciation for "giftedness." He also seems to think that the pursuit of enhancements will lead to loss of the sense of giftedness, so he has consequentialist concerns as well. The sense of giftedness, according to Sandel, includes an acceptance of the limitations of human powers and an "openness to the unbidden," to what we cannot control. Sandel also asserts that the sense of "giftedness" is a precondition for having proper humility and perhaps other virtues as well.[8]

Given how highly he esteems the sense of "giftedness" and given that he refrains from considering whether there is any combination of other goods that enhancement might provide which could compensate for a diminution of the sense of "giftedness," it seems plausible to think that Sandel rejects what I called in Chapter Two the Balancing Approach to the ethics of enhancement.[9] In other words, if one takes the giftedness argument at face value, its conclusion appears to be that the enhancement enterprise is *ipso facto* such an assault on central human values that any attempt to appraise the pros and cons of enhancement reveals a kind of moral obtuseness. On this view, we *already* know enough about enhancement to conclude that it is a bad thing; we need not trouble ourselves with canvassing all the pros and cons and then trying, somehow, to come to an all-things-considered judgment. So Sandel's giftedness argument could be interpreted as showing that the Balancing Approach I am advocating is radically misconceived.

One virtue of understanding Sandel's argument in this way is that it explains something about his work that is otherwise very puzzling: the fact that he never seriously considers the benefits of enhancement, nor asks whether they could outweigh whatever threat to the virtue of "giftedness" enhancement poses. There are, of course, other explanations of this feature of his work. For example, perhaps he is a polemicist, rather than an ethicist committed to trying to achieve an even-handed treatment of the issues. My interpretation is more charitable and that is a good reason to pursue it.

I now want to show that Sandel's reflections on "giftedness" do not support the conclusion that we should reject the Balancing Approach. I will also argue that they do not support a rejection of enhancement across the board or of the enhancement enterprise. I begin with an attempt to translate Sandel's rhetoric about giftedness into an argument.

1. The sense of the giftedness is a central human good (or an important aspect of good character).

2. The drive for mastery is incompatible with the sense of giftedness.

3. The employment of biomedical enhancements is an instance of the drive for mastery.

4. (Therefore) the employment of biomedical enhancements is incompatible with the sense of giftedness.

5. Therefore, the employment of biomedical enhancements is incompatible with a central human good.

As it stands, even if this very bold argument were sound, it would not show that the Balancing Approach is wrong, because it leaves open the possibility that there might be some good or combination of goods that can only be attained by biomedical enhancement that would compensate for the loss of the central good of the sense of "giftedness." If this were the case, then it would be perfectly appropriate to try to take these other goods into account as reasons for enhancement. Suppose, then, that one grants Sandel an additional premise:

6. If something is incompatible with a central human good, then this incompatibility is a conclusive reason against it.

7. Therefore, there is a conclusive reason against biomedical enhancement (and we need not consider the "pros" of biomedical enhancement).

This sixth premise is far from self-evident. Perhaps human life is tragic: not all of the most important goods are compatible. Even if one

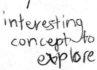
interesting
concept to
explore

grants the sixth premise to Sandel, however, the argument still fails. The most obvious problem is the falsity of premise 3: people can and do coherently pursue enhancements of many different sorts, including biomedical enhancements, without exhibiting a "drive for mastery" that is incompatible with any sense of giftedness that could plausibly be construed as a central human good. In other words, premise 3 is a false generalization that overlooks the complexity of human motivation; and, in any event, Sandel does nothing whatsoever to provide evidence to support it.

Here are two of many examples to make the falsity of premise 3 crystal clear. Suppose that I am having laser surgery on my eyes to correct myopia. I opt for overcorrection, for better than 20/20 vision, because this will enhance my bird-watching ability on those occasions on which my binoculars are not at hand. Have I thereby exhibited a desire for mastery? No: the desire for having to rely on my binoculars a little less often for satisfactory bird-watching is not a desire for mastery by any stretch of the imagination; to say that it is would be irresponsible hyperbole. In opting for some over correction, do I *thereby* reveal a lack of an appropriate sense of giftedness? Obviously not. Opting for over-correction is no evidence whatsoever that I fail to appreciate that much of what is good in life is not subject to human control. Similarly, if one pursues cognitive—as opposed to visual—biomedical enhancements, whether as individuals or as a matter of social investment in increased productivity, does this show a desire for mastery that is incompatible with a sense of giftedness that qualifies for being a central human good? If the answer to this question is yes—and surely it is *not*—then literacy, numeracy, immunization, and the use of computers are all profound moral wrongs—and that central human good, the sense of giftedness, was wantonly destroyed long ago. Sandel's warning that one should not imperil the sense of "giftedness" comes several millennia too late. Remember: Sandel has given us no reason to think that the mere fact that an enhancement involves biomedical means shows that the pursuit of it betrays a craving for mastery or perfection. Instead, he is committed to the patently false view that the pursuit of any enhancement, whether biomedical or not, betrays such unseemly motivation, and that is clearly false. In fact, it is so clearly false that it is hard to know which is more puzzling: the fact that Sandel makes such a claim or the fact that some people have taken it seriously.

It is also crucial to understand that Sandel does not restrict his claims about mastery and giftedness to efforts to enhance children—his opposition is to enhancement as such. Even if he did it would still be unsound. The fact that one immunizes one's child, or provides her with an education, a computer, or other cognitive enhancements is in itself no evidence whatsoever that one desires to master the conditions of its existence or that one is not "open" to appreciation of features of one's child's existence that one cannot control. To assume that the pursuit of biomedical enhancements, unlike the pursuit of these more familiar enhancements, betrays a craving for mastery or a lack of appreciation for giftedness is to beg the question and to be guilty of biomedical enhancement exceptionalism. The mere fact that an enhancement is biomedical could not make its pursuit motivationally tainted.

Now consider a much more dramatic enhancement: a significant extension of the typical human lifespan, say to 400 years. We could succeed in achieving this enhancement for all human beings and yet not be under the delusion that we have achieved mastery of the conditions of our lives or of the attributes of our children—unless we were remarkably blind to the nature of human existence. In a society in which the lifespan was 400 years, there would still be plenty of things to sustain the sense of "giftedness." People would still die of accidents; wars presumably would still occur; deadly pandemics presumably would still arise; people would still fall in love with people who do not love them and fail in every effort to make themselves loveable; children would still sometimes wound their parents by repudiating their values or failing to appreciate their sacrifices; people would still invest in careers and projects that fail, despite the best laid plans; the weather and natural disasters, would still be beyond our control; many human actions, both individual and collective, would still have unpredicted consequences, etc., etc.

Whenever individuals did *not* suffer such misfortunes, they would have occasion for the sense of giftedness, for an appreciation that many of the most important goods humans enjoy, including life itself, are not within their control and never will be. There would still be countless positive reasons for appreciating the giftedness of human life: the good fortune of having met one's soul mate, of having had the opportunity to be a part of an important social movement because one was born at the right time, of having read a particular book at just the right time in one's life for it to make an impact on one's character, of having chosen a career that turns out to be socially valued, of having children who grow up to be good people, and so forth. Opportunities for a sense of "giftedness" would not be lacking in a world replete with biomedical enhancements. Contrary to Sandel, in such a world it would not be the case that "there would be nothing left to affirm or behold outside our own will."[10] A world in which every society whole-heartedly engaged in the enhancement project would not be a world from which contingency was banished. Can one really imagine a headline like this: "Harvard Professor Predicts Contingency Shortage; Stock Market Plummets"?

It is difficult to understand how Sandel could think that even universal employment of the most extreme biomedical enhancements would make much of a dent in the lack of control that characterizes so much of the good and the bad in human life, how he could believe that even the widespread use of biomedical enhancements could banish chance and reduce everything to human choice. Could he really believe what he says when he asserts that if we pursue enhancements we will traverse a slippery slope whose terminus is a world in which "there would be nothing left to affirm or behold outside our own will"? Ironically, if Sandel means what he says, it is he who has an inadequate appreciation of the giftedness of human life—and a vastly inflated conception of biomedical empowerment. Only a genetic determinist on steroids (so to speak) would think that even the most thorough-going pursuit of perfection through biotechnology could banish contingency from human life and rob us of ample opportunities for exhibiting the sense of "giftedness."

Sandel might reply indignantly that I have misinterpreted him. His claim about "there being nothing left to . . . behold outside our own will" is not meant to be taken at face value. He does not really mean, contrary to what he says, that enhancements would destroy the sense of giftedness by eliminating our lack of control over the good things in life (leaving us with nothing to contemplate but our own will). Rather, his point is that the pursuit of enhancements is likely to *diminish* our precious sense of giftedness.

Given how much there is in life to prompt the sense of giftedness—given how extensive the domain of contingency is—it is hard to know what would count as a significant diminution of our sense of giftedness, much less such a *dangerous* diminution as to warrant forgoing all of the goods that some biomedical enhancements would bring. Given the ubiquity of lack of control in human life, and the imperviousness of so much of it to biomedical enhancements, is humanity really threatened with a giftedness shortage? Is it likely that biomedical enhancements will reduce the domain humans cannot control to the point that our sense of giftedness will be too weak for us to have a good life? What reason is there to believe that there is such a threshold or that we are likely to approach it? Sandel does not say. I cannot imagine what he could plausibly say.

Consider yet another interpretation of Sandel's argument. Perhaps his point is not that we are in danger of a shortage of lack of control—and an ensuing sense-of-giftedness shortage—but rather that pursuing enhancements will cause us to come to *believe* that we can master the conditions of human existence—and that this *belief* will cause us to lose the sense of giftedness. If this is his argument, then he is resting the case against enhancement on a very strong prediction that pursuing enhancement will cause a delusion of such proportions as to be tantamount to collective madness. Yet he provides no evidence for the hypothesis that enhancements will cause such a delusion. Sandel's references to cases of "hyper-parenting" certainly do not supply the needed evidence. It is one thing to say that people, or some people, may overdo enhancements, quite another to say that a significant number of people will become so deeply deluded as to think that they are or could be masters of the human condition.

Another interpretation may be worth considering. Perhaps Sandel's remarks about giftedness are intended simply as a reminder that the possibility of enhancement may, for some people, provide a new outlet for unsavory tendencies they already have, including an overestimation of their ability to control things. If that is his point, it is hardly a new one. It has been the stock and trade of critics of technology for at least a couple of hundred years and it reveals nothing peculiar to biomedical enhancements. More importantly, that familiar reminder falls far short of rejecting the Balancing Approach or of providing an argument against biomedical enhancement across the board or for not embarking on the enhancement enterprise. In fact, it is hard to see what its practical implications are.

In fairness to Sandel, perhaps I should consider one last, even more deflationary interpretation of his giftedness "argument." Perhaps Sandel is only saying that if humans pursue enhancement *without limit*, they thereby exhibit a drive for mastery that is incompatible with a virtuous or good human life. On this interpretation, the only practical import of the giftedness argument is a warning not to pursue enhancements without limit, not to strive for perfection as opposed to improvement, along with some anecdotes that are supposed to show that Americans— or is it upper-middle-class Americans?—have dispositions that exacerbate the risk of doing so. Again, this is hardly novel, much less earthshaking. After all, pursuing virtually anything without limit is a bad idea and we've known that for some time. On this interpretation, as with all the others, the giftedness argument provides nothing approaching a conclusive reason against biomedical enhancement across the board or a good reason for not pursuing the enhancement enterprise. Whether the enhancement enterprise is a good idea depends not only on how the expected benefits of enhancement stack up against the risk that it will exacerbate some people's excessive desire for control, but also on whether we can devise effective ways of restraining the tendency toward inappropriate attempts at mastery.

— we don't act like we know that - not sure if ever7 know that

Sandel is to be commended for calling to our attention to some considerations that should be taken into account in doing the hard work of identifying and trying to balance the pros and cons of various enhancements. On the stronger and more interesting interpretations, his reflections on giftedness are remarkably implausible. On the weaker interpretation they are familiar, even commonsensical, but of limited value in helping us determine what we should do about enhancement. Contrary to his claim in *Against Perfection*, he has not provided an "argument against enhancement."

Nevertheless, there may be other ways to spell out character concerns, and some of them may bear some important relationship to concerns about an excessive desire for mastery or a failure to appreciate the given. In the remainder of this chapter, I distinguish and try to evaluate three concerns that meet this description.

"Gratitude" and the appreciation of existing goods

Some critics of enhancement say that there is a connection between the desire for biomedical enhancements and a failure to exhibit the virtue of gratitude. I want to explore this idea, while avoiding two errors that I have already pointed out: assuming that anyone who desires

Gratitude: "The quality of being thankful"
Thankful: "pleased & relieved"
Pleased: "feeling or showing pleasure & satisfacti
especially at an event or situation"

enhancement thereby betrays an unseemly craving for mastery (or for perfection), and taking the term "gratitude" at face value rather than treating it as a clumsy stand-in for something more apt and less encumbered by theological baggage. My suggestion is quite simple: we *should* be concerned about the risk that we will become so focused on the improvements that we can attain through biomedical means that we will fail to show proper appreciation for the goods we already have. After explaining just why we should be worried about this, I will attempt to do what critics of enhancement usually fail to do: determine the practical implications of taking this worry seriously.

Let us begin by focusing on the virtue of *appreciation*. The notion of appreciation actually serves the purposes of critics of enhancement better than that of gratitude, at least if they wish to make a case against enhancement that does not depend on disputed religious premises. "Appreciation," unlike "gratitude," does not imply that the good to be appreciated is the result of an agent's action. People who either do not hold religious views of the sort that could ground gratitude, or who believe that public discourse about enhancement should not invoke such views, can grasp the importance of the virtue of gratitude. In addition, as I will show, whatever is of value in talk about gratitude in this context can be captured just as well by relying on the less problematic notion of appreciation.

gratitude doesn't do that

In exploring the virtue of appreciation and its relevance to practical questions about biomedical enhancement, we will be venturing into the domain of Conservatism as a moral–political point of view. In Chapter Five I examine in greater detail the implications of Conservatism for enhancement—and vice versa. Here I only want to note that the virtue of appreciation plays a central role in Conservative thought. Please note that by "Conservatism," I do not mean what some Americans call Conservatism, namely, the view that "government is the problem not the solution," and that the US should take what is euphemistically called a "forward leaning" posture when it comes to using its military assets in the pursuit of foreign policy. Instead, I am concerned with Conservatism as a more nuanced tradition in moral–political thought that traces its pedigree back at least to the thinking of Edmund Burke in the late eighteenth century.

Conservatism emphasizes the importance of enjoying and valuing the good things that now exist, where this entails taking pains to preserve them, including the cultivation of a presumption against endangering them through the pursuit of novelty or even of things thought to have greater value.[11] To understand the significance of this key conservative insight, it is useful to distinguish several distinct reasons in support of a bias toward existing goods. First, and most obviously, our lives can go less well when we restlessly pursue improvement at the expense of a proper appreciation of the goods we now possess. This is the stuff of films and novels. To be constantly focused on future goods is to be distracted from the enjoyment of existing goods, and although enjoyment is not the sum total of human well-being, it is a prominent ingredient therein.

agreed

Consider, for example, the predicament of Julien Sorel in Stendhal's profoundly ironic, proto-existentialist novel, *The Red and the Black*, to which Camus' *The Stranger* owes so much. Julien is deprived of happiness, even as he attains his most cherished goals, because his ceaselessly strategic, calculating behavior—his relentless focus on how to attain his next "victory"—prevents him from enjoying what he achieves. Failure to appreciate the value of what already exists and hence the importance of sustaining it can also lead to another kind of loss, as when a person who strives to make more friends neglects and eventually loses the friends she has.

Second, a person who constantly focuses on how to achieve new goods at the expense of the enjoyment of those she already possesses betrays a character flaw. She is insufficiently appreciative of her good fortune. This is the vice of greediness, of immoderate appetite or insatiability.

true

Third, to the extent that the good things we now possess are the result of the labors and struggles of past generations, a failure to appreciate them properly is a failure to esteem those people, to value duly their accomplishments and the sacrifices they made to achieve them. In extreme cases, this arguably amounts to wronging them.

Fourth, if people's interests can survive them in the sense that they have an interest in states of affairs that will exist after their own deaths, then there can be cases in which a readiness to risk existing goods for the sake of new ones can constitute a failure to take the interests of other persons seriously. For example, if the current generation of a certain community decides to change the community's constitution without taking seriously the fact that in doing so they will thwart the interests

[handwritten margin note top: meh? Kind of blurry. We don't owe our predecessors the act of carrying out their virtues or intentions. What if we disagree w them?]

of their predecessors in creating and sustaining a certain kind of community, they act wrongly.

[handwritten left margin: failing to understand it or just seeking it]

Finally, in some cases, pursuing new goods to the detriment of existing ones may be a personal betrayal that signals a lack of understanding of the nature of the most valuable relationships. This would occur, for example, if a person abandoned her friend or lover simply for the sake of the opportunity to gain a new one who better satisfied her needs and desires. Such a person, as G.A. Cohen puts it, would make the mistake of trying to maximize value at the expense of failing to appreciate what has value, but she would also be guilty of being disloyal or of failing to understand what love or friendship is.[12] For all of these reasons, cultivating a presumption in favor of existing goods, that is, a presumption against efforts to improve that imperil existing goods, seems appropriate.

[handwritten left margin: Is this because it's simply the "opportunity to do so and not a given therefore you may end up with neither the original friend or the new one?]

But what are the practical implications of this conclusion? The difficulty is that a completely general, that is, *nondiscriminating* presumption against efforts to improve would clearly be irrational, because it would preclude any progress whatsoever, whether personal or social. The alternative would be to cultivate a discriminating presumption— a presumption in favor of *some* existing goods or types of existing goods, where these goods are to be identified in some principled way. Clearly, we would need an account of how this principled identification is to be achieved. One suspects that most of the heavy moral lifting would have to be done at this stage, in the effort to determine just when we ought to forgo efforts at improvement and rest content with existing goods. If that is the case, then the idea of the virtue of appreciation does not get us very far. But quite apart from that, cultivating and sustaining a complex, discriminating presumption in favor of existing goods may be very difficult, at least for many people, given current cognitive and motivational limitations. In contrast, a highly general, nondiscriminating, presumption in favor of the status quo might be more socially and psychologically feasible, but such a presumption appears to be incapable of plausibly ruling out anything as multifaceted as the enhancement project.

The threads of the argument can now be pulled together. The pursuit of enhancements, for some individuals, in some circumstances, might both express and exacerbate a tendency to fail to appreciate and enjoy the goods they now have in their rush to attain new goods. Depending on the circumstances, this error could merely be a case of imprudence or self-thwarting behavior, or it could be an injustice to others, a personal betrayal, a misunderstanding of the nature of love or friendship, a lack of appreciation of good fortune, or an instance of greediness and insatiability. Further, once we appreciate the circumstances in which biomedical enhancements are likely to become available, the Conservative admonition to appreciate the goods we now possess becomes all the more important, because powerful marketing forces, including the ubiquitous promptings of mass culture, may worsen the tendency to undervalue what we have in the pursuit of what we lack.

Nevertheless, due regard for the virtue of appreciation cannot provide a good reason for refraining from biomedical enhancements across the board, anymore than it can provide a good reason for a wholesale rejection of other attempts to improve human or personal well-being. Any presumption in favor of existing goods robust and general enough to rule out biomedical enhancement across the board would block off too many avenues of progress. For example, it would presumably rule out the invention of literacy, agriculture, science, and market economies, since each of these developments creates a risk that some people—perhaps many people—will focus excessively on future improvements at the cost of failing to appreciate fully what they already have.

[margin note: very ~much something present today]

Moreover, if the benefits of particular enhancements are great enough, then the cost of avoiding the tendency to undervalue existing goods by refraining from the enhancement project will be unacceptably high, especially if there are other less extreme precautions we can take to counteract this tendency. Further, a proper presumption in favor of existing goods cannot rule out enhancements in circumstances in which enhancements are needed *to preserve existing things we rightly cherish.* In Chapters One and Two, I explored briefly the idea that enhancements may be needed to preserve present levels of well-being, not just to attain higher ones. (Recall Tancredi, in *The Leopard*, who sagely observes that to keep things the same, things will need to change.[13]) In Chapter Five I probe this possibility further.

[margin note: ~ something to ponder]

Even if due regard for the virtue of appreciation does not rule out enhancements across the board, does it provide a strong reason against embarking on the enhancement enterprise? The answer to that question is harder to ascertain. It depends on whether we are more likely to sustain a proper appreciation of existing goods if we face the inevitable emergence of biomedical enhancements head-on—that is, by trying to subject them to constraints developed in the light of public deliberations and democratic political processes within a constitutional order of entrenched individual rights, rather than simply allowing them to come in the back door. It also depends on whether we can improve—by biomedical or other means—either our capacity for appreciating existing goods or our capacity to act consistently on that appreciation.

It is *possible* that the risk of worsening the tendency toward the under-appreciation of existing goods will be increased if we embark on the enhancement enterprise instead of simply continuing to allow enhancements to emerge helter-skelter as spin-offs from efforts to treat and prevent disease. It *might* turn out that the risk of excessive preoccupation with improvement increases with the availability of biomedical enhancements, and that there will be greater availability if the enhancement project is pursued than if it is not. But even if we assume that all of this is the case, it is important to emphasize that whether this added risk amounts to a conclusive reason against embarking on the enhancement enterprise depends crucially upon whether the benefits that the enhancement project would bring outweigh those added risks.

In my judgment, a proper regard for the virtue of appreciation at present does not provide a conclusive reason against undertaking the enhancement project. It might turn out, however, that as the enhancement enterprise unfolds, we will learn that whatever benefits enhancements are bringing are outweighed by the loss of well-being we suffer from constantly being focused on new enhancements. *Taking that possibility seriously may speak in favor of the enhancement enterprise rather than against it, however, if our chances for accurately evaluating the fruits of enhancement and taking a more restrained posture toward it are increased by making enhancement a legitimate social goal, subject to monitoring, public deliberation, and regulation.*

Perhaps in the end the greatest strength of the concern about gratitude—or more accurately, about appreciation—is that it urges us to take seriously the crucial point, already noted in Chapter One, that an enhancement need not bring an increase in well-being. Julian Savulescu has suggested to me that perhaps the core idea is that a good life is one in which a person concentrates on making the best of what she has been given, where this includes duly appreciating the goods she possesses. One is reminded of Thurgood Marshall's statement that he hoped that

agree w/ this idea

people would recognize that "he did the best he could with what he had to work with."

The difficulty with Savulescu's suggestion is, I hope, now a familiar one: it is hard to know what its practical implications for enhancement are. If the claim is that we should always accept our current limitations and focus only on the goods we have, it is clearly indefensible. Sometimes enhancing some of our capacities does increase our well-being overall. And it is not hard to think of situations in which undertaking a biomedical enhancement, rather than simply resting content with the status quo would be the only way to prevent a serious *decrease* in a person's well-being.

Consider the following case. John is a person who has always been athletic. His well-being depends very substantially on his capacity for engaging in vigorous, physically demanding sports. On due reflection, and in the light of an accurate appraisal of his own psychology, John concludes that as he advances into old age he will not be able to participate or at least participate well enough in vigorous sports to derive much enjoyment from them. He reasonably predicts a significant decrease in his well-being. He decides that it would be better, from the standpoint of his personal well-being, if he were to begin to cultivate the capacity for more sedentary enjoyments—activities he will be able to engage when his days as an athlete come to an end. He envies people who take great pleasure from long sessions of listening to music or sitting on benches in museums contemplating great works of art. He believes, quite reasonably, that "what he was given"—his natural endowment—is a capacity to derive well-being from vigorous sports activities and that his "natural" capacity for more sedentary enjoyments is quite meager. He tries very hard to develop his capacity for enjoying sedentary activities, but makes little progress. Then he learns that his efforts to cultivate the capacity for sedentary enjoyments will be much more likely to succeed if he takes a particular drug. It could be a drug for attention deficit disorder, such as Ritalin; or it could be a new drug that enhances the functioning of the brain in processing auditory stimuli, with the effect that it makes one better able to discriminate nuances in music, while at the same time increasing the release of endorphins that tend to occur at high levels in people whose natural endowment includes a keen appreciation for music. Under these circumstances, John will do better, from the standpoint of personal well-being, if he undertakes an

good example

enhancement than if he follows the advice of making the best of what he has. In fact, if his capacity for enjoying vigorous sports diminishes or disappears altogether and he does not develop alternative modes of enjoyment, his well-being will decline significantly from its present level.

The point of this example is not to deny that it is often good advice to make the best of what one has. The point, rather, is that this generally sound counsel admits of many exceptions, in life generally, and perhaps especially in a world in which biomedical enhancements are increasingly available. Notice also that the well-being John will enjoy if he undertakes the enhancement is not pseudo-happiness or passive enjoyment—the enhancement will simply enable him to engage in *activities* that will require the exercise of skills, effort, etc. This is not the "soma" of *Brave New World*.

The preceding paragraph merely scratches the surface of a deep and complex topic: the relationship between the natural or what is "given" to us by nature and well-being. In the next chapter I explore this relationship much more thoroughly. At this point, I simply want to note that the example of John, the aging athlete, shows that it is *not* always true that we do best from the standpoint of personal well-being by merely working with what we are "given."

Self-manipulation/objectification

I now turn to another worry about enhancement that may not fit as comfortably under the heading of character concerns as the idea that enhancement betrays an unseemly craving for mastery or perfection or a lack of appreciation for existing good. Nevertheless, I think this concern may lie beneath the rhetoric about the pursuit of perfection and the craving for mastery. What I have in mind is the evocative but murky charge that the use of biomedical enhancements betrays a profoundly mistaken—and demeaning—attitude toward the self, namely, that it is an object to be manipulated. Perhaps the *locus classicus* of this concern is the work of Martin Heidegger.[14] Whether or not this worry is properly described as a concern about character, it has something in common with the character concerns already considered: it is an attempt to show that the pursuit of enhancements involves distorted values or serious moral misperceptions.

As a first step toward understanding and evaluating the concern about self-objectification/manipulation, I will make what may initially seem to be an outrageous claim: *not only is nothing wrong* per se *with regarding oneself as an object or with manipulating oneself, but also there are cases in which it is morally obligatory to do so.* To understand this fundamental point, consider cases of rational *self-binding.* The paradigm of self-binding is the behavior of Ulysses: he has his men bind him to the mast and stuff wax in their ears, as the ship passes near the island of the Sirens. Ulysses recognizes that he is imperfectly rational—that if he is able to do so he will respond to the Sirens' song, in spite of his knowledge that to do so means death. He also has a desire to hear the Sirens' song. He uses his rationality to have it both ways: to be able to hear the Sirens' song but not be killed. His rational strategy for coping with his imperfect rationality is to restrict his options: by being bound to the mast, he does not have the option of jumping ship and swimming to the Sirens.

Restricting options is only one of many ways of using one's reason to cope with one's imperfect rationality. Another is to subject oneself to a cost or penalty if one fails to follow through on a decision. The late Joel Feinberg once told me that he made a vow in front of his students that he was quitting smoking, because he knew that his desire to avoid the shame of their seeing him fail to follow through would help him stick to his resolve. A friend of mine who was having trouble finishing his dissertation used another strategy: he signed a contract with a behavioral therapist. If he failed to produce five pages of dissertation work a week, the therapist would mail a check signed by my friend to a religious group that he abhorred. (He never failed to meet his writing quota.)

The incentives one creates to cope with one's imperfect rationality can be positive as well as negative: many of us motivate ourselves to do things we know we should do but find it difficult to do, by setting up rewards. We use our rationality to set up conditions that will cause us to act rationally, in spite of our propensity for acting irrationally.

In all of these cases of rationally coping with imperfect rationality, we regard ourselves as objects, and as targets of manipulation, in this straightforward sense: we step back and see ourselves as predictably subject to causal influences and then subject ourselves to particular causal influences that will enable us to do what we would otherwise be unable to do. To put the point a bit more crudely: we temporarily dissociate from ourselves as subjects so as to consider ourselves as objects, as reasonably reliable machines that convert certain inputs into outputs. Let us call this "rational self-manipulation." The point is that rational self-manipulation essentially involves treating the self as an object and that there is nothing wrong with it *per se*.

To cope with our imperfect rationality, we must regard ourselves as *less than* pure subjects whose will is always sufficient for producing the behavior we choose. In other words, to acknowledge our imperfect rationality is to admit that to a degree we are like objects, things subject to external causal influences that can thwart our practical rationality. In some cases, our self-manipulation/objectification is not merely a matter of achieving what we happen to prefer: we are morally obligated to avoid foreseeable weakness of the will by subjecting ourselves to appropriate incentives or, as in the case of Ulysses-like self-binding, taking certain options off the table pre-emptively. For example, a person who has good reason to believe that when he inherits a large fortune he will neglect his duties of charity, might sign a legal instrument that would pre-authorize dispensing some of the funds he will inherit to certain designated charities. Similarly, a person who knows that she is at risk for being unfaithful to her spouse if she contacts a previous partner might deliberately delete the latter's email address and phone number from her records.

Rational self-manipulation for moral purposes need not be confined to foreclosing options, as in self-binding cases. Sometimes, especially strong emotions can restrict our options, including the option of doing the right thing, because they impair our judgment. In these cases, we might enhance our moral capacity by moderating the emotions in question so as to increase, not limit, our options.[15] For example, if we are prone to extreme anger toward those who disagree with us on certain political issues, this anger may prevent us from seeing that there are possibilities for morally acceptable compromises.

The argument thus far can be succinctly summarized. Coping with our imperfect rationality, at least in cases in which we do so by subjecting ourselves to positive or negative incentives, *essentially* involves treating ourselves as objects to be manipulated. But clearly there are many cases in which it is not only permissible, but even morally obligatory, to cope with our imperfect rationality. Therefore, *treating ourselves as objects to be manipulated cannot in itself be wrong*. So, if there is something wrong with biomedical enhancements, it cannot be (simply) that they involve self-objectification/manipulation.

What we need, of course, is a distinction between *appropriately* and *inappropriately* treating ourselves as objects to be manipulated. Kant tells us that we should never treat a person (including ourselves) as a *mere* means; he does not say, and should not say, that it is never permissible to treat a person as a means. The crucial question is this: Under what conditions and for what reasons is it morally permissible (or even obligatory) to treat oneself as an object of manipulation? Part of the answer to this question, following Kant, is that we must not treat ourselves as if we were mere things, rather than beings with a good of their own and a capacity for practical rationality.

Notice that it will not do to reply that when we cope with our imperfect rationality by *biomedical* means we thereby inappropriately treat ourselves as objects to be manipulated and fail to acknowledge our status as persons, not mere things. That would be biomedical exceptionalism, pure and simple, and it would beg the very question at issue, namely, whether, or in what conditions, employing biomedical enhancements is compatible with a proper attitude of respect toward oneself. Once we acknowledge, as we must, that there is nothing wrong with rational self-manipulation *per se*, the burden of argument rests instead on someone who claims that there is something especially morally problematic about rational self-manipulation by biomedical means.

I can think of no reason to think that biomedical rational self-manipulation is especially morally problematic, from the standpoint of avoiding the error or of treating oneself as a mere means. Nor are biomedical means unique in constraining our freedom of action or in operating without our conscious direction, once the choice to use them has been made—the same is true with traditional self-binding techniques.

It may turn out, however, that there are *other* ways in which rational self-manipulation can go wrong besides by treating oneself as a mere means. And, for all we know at this point in the investigation, rational self-manipulation that involves biomedical means may be more prone to these errors.

To explore that possibility, I propose a strategy: let us try to sort out the chief moral risks of rational self-manipulation and then see whether they are especially great in the case of uses of biomedical enhancements that qualify as rational self-manipulation. There are at least three moral risks that warrant our attention: (1) atrophy of the moral powers, (2) loss of spontaneity, and (3) lack of proper appreciation for existing goods. I have already explored (3) in some detail and will continue to do so in Chapter Five, so here I will concentrate on the other two. In each case, the task will be to try to assess the moral risk we are likely to face in a world in which biomedical technologies increase our opportunities for treating ourselves—or, more accurately, treating some of our character-istics—as "objects" upon which we can exert causal influences. Proceed-ing in this way will further my strategy of trying to extract the grains of truth embedded in unsatisfyingly vague (and hyperbolic) rhetoric about perfection, the craving for mastery, and lack of "gratitude."

Atrophy of the moral powers

The worry here is most pronounced in the opposition to performance-enhancing drugs in sports, but it applies to other enhancement contexts as well. The idea is that if we can get a biomedical "quick fix" for our problems, we will not be forced to exercise our willpower and that disuse will produce atrophy. In its most general form, this concern cannot provide a conclusive reason against enhancements, for a fairly obvious reason: sometimes what we gain from a technology is worth the weak-ening of the natural capacities it improves upon. For example, it may well be the case that the increasing use of GPS devices has led, or will eventually lead, to a decline in traditional orientation skills on the part of hikers, hunters, woodsmen, and the average automobile driver. But from this it doesn't follow that we should abandon our GPS devices, much less that reliance on them is a vice. So even if reliance on a technology results in the atrophying of a skill or capacity, it doesn't follow that it is wrong to rely on it.

It is important not to confuse two distinct judgments about technolog-ical shortcuts: judgments about whether they are permissible and judg-ments about whether employing them is *less good* in *some respect* than attaining the same goals without the shortcuts. It might be true that it is *better* to get to one's destination by exercising traditional orientation skills than simply consulting a GPS, in this sense: if you get there the old-fashioned way, you merit commendation for possessing a fairly complex skill, the development of which usually takes considerable effort. But from this it doesn't follow that it is *wrong* to use a GPS.[16] Life is not a contest in which the goal is to do everything in the most difficult way. *Moral powers* are different from orienteering skills, one might protest! That is not so obvious, however. Traditional moral education involves "technologies," such as rule-following (and, on some accounts, deference to religious authority), that are designed to *replace* moral deliberation about particular matters.

Sometimes such rules are reliable proxies for deliberation when there is no time for deliberation; in other cases, their use enables us to avoid errors of deliberation that are likely to occur when emotions run high or when temptations are especially strong. To the extent that we come to rely on general moral rules, our powers of deliberating about the nuances of particular moral situations may deteriorate, but some deterioration may be worthwhile, all things considered. The ideal moral education would strike a balance between reliance on rules (or authorities) and particularized moral deliberation. In the economist's terms, the problem is one of optimizing, not maximizing either reliance on rules or case-by-case, detailed deliberation. Given our imperfect rationality and the limits of our information, any balance we strike, any trade-off we make between the two values, will carry risks. The risk of atrophy of the moral powers is one of those risks. This is a general point about reliance on technologies, not one that is peculiar to biomedical technologies or to biomedical enhancement technologies. It is no more capable of grounding a conclusion that we should eschew biomedical enhancements than a conclusion that we should abandon technologies generally.

So far I have been indulging in a simplification, by proceeding as if the idea of the atrophying of the moral powers was transparent and unproblematic. It is not, as the following example illustrates. Recent scientific studies indicate that resisting temptations is morally fatiguing, and that as with vigorous exercise, there is a recovery period during which one's moral reserves are depleted.[17] The same studies suggest that a simple biochemical intervention—ingesting glucose—can shorten the recovery period. The brain runs on glucose. Perhaps adding glucose speeds the recovery of full functioning in the brain centers involved in resisting temptations.

Suppose that these findings become well confirmed and are put into practice on a large scale. People facing morally strenuous situations take a glucose pill in advance, in order to increase the probability that they will do the right thing. In one perfectly straightforward sense, the practice of "moral glucose-loading" would be an *increase* in our moral powers, not an atrophying of them: we would still have to exert will power, but we would have a greater capacity to withstand temptations, because our moral recovery time from exertions of the will would be shorter.

In the scenario I have just described, there is no apparent risk that our moral powers will become atrophied. But even if there were such a risk, it would not follow that we should not avail ourselves of this enhancement. That would depend upon whether the moral benefits of the enhancement outweighed the risk of atrophy. To put the same point differently: some diminution of one moral capacity might be a price worth paying if the gain in some other moral capacity were great enough.

Consider a final twist on the thought experiment: suppose that the substance that increased our moral capacity in this way were not glucose, but instead some new molecule invented in the laboratory. Would this make a moral difference? Presumably it would not. To say that self-manipulation for the sake of better moral conduct is permissible when it utilizes the "natural" substance glucose, but impermissible when it uses "artificial" or man-made substances, would make sense only if the concept of the natural were capable of doing a great deal of moral work. In the next chapter, I argue that it is not.

Another point about the moral atrophy worry is worth making. Recall that this worry is voiced most strongly in the case of performance-enhancing drugs in sports. Ironically, it appears to be quite misplaced even in that context, at least if we attend to what really goes on when serious athletes use such drugs. Using "blood-doping" or anabolic steroids does not replace effort; it enables athletes to train even harder, by allowing their bodies to recover more quickly from punishing exercise regimens. There is no evidence that athletes who use performance-enhancing drugs train less rigorously or exert less effort to excel.

Loss of spontaneity

A person who obsessively focuses on constantly improving himself, whether by biomedical or more traditional means, runs the risk of losing an important ingredient of a good human life: spontaneity. Again,

Stendhal's character Julien Sorel provides a vivid illustration. Julien lives constantly in the forward-looking, calculating, strategic mode. He treats himself as an instrument for achieving his strategic goals. The result is that his life is almost devoid of spontaneity. (Ironically, in the only instance in which he exhibits spontaneous emotion, the result is that he attains something he has not been able to achieve by cold calculated action— the seduction of Madame de Renal.) A good human life includes more than calculated, deliberate action. It includes considerable scope for spontaneity: for acting on impulse, following one's feelings, going with the flow, not always being in charge, and just *having* emotions rather than deliberately inducing them.

It is not hard to see that there are connections among the worries about mastery, perfectionism, lack of appreciation of the good, inappropriate self-manipulation, and loss of spontaneity. A life in which one was constantly pursuing new enhancement, out of an overweening desire for mastery or perfection, would exhibit a lack of appreciation for the goods one already has, would involve treating oneself as a mere instrument for attaining improvements, and would also be lacking in spontaneity.

To a greater or lesser degree, there are already people who fit this description and presumably there always have been, at least wherever people have managed to do more than subsist. In a culture like ours, the risk of falling into an obsession with improvement that gives short shrift to spontaneity is heightened by the pressures of mass media advertising. If a broad panoply of biomedical enhancements becomes available and affordable, the problem may be exacerbated.

The question we must ask once again is: "So what?" Does it follow that we should try to forgo biomedical enhancements or, if that is impossible, as seems likely, that we should at least refrain from engaging in the enhancement enterprise? Or is the point that we must somehow engage in that enterprise in a way that reduces the risk of loss of spontaneity; and, if so, how might we do that? Recall that the proper question to ask is whether embracing the enhancement project will produce a greater risk of loss of spontaneity than allowing biomedical enhancements to develop willy-nilly, entering through the backdoor of treatment and prevention research—*not* whether it will produce a greater risk of loss of spontaneity than a world without biomedical enhancements.

The issue is not whether the availability of biomedical enhancements will result in a risk of loss of spontaneity, but whether it will result in an *unacceptable* risk of loss of spontaneity. (After all, most worthwhile things involve risk) Whether the risk is unacceptable will depend upon several factors, but two are perhaps especially important: cost and moral restraint. If biomedical enhancements are costly enough, then an unending quest for improvement through their utilization will be beyond the reach of all but the wealthiest. High cost can even reduce the demand for highly addictive substances: cigarette sales go down when they are taxed heavily.

I argued in Chapter One that we should not assume that biomedical enhancements will remain very costly, so we cannot assume that this constraint will be effective. One option would be to adopt policies that deliberately increase the cost of (some) biomedical enhancements. The major drawback to this strategy, of course, is that it has the features of a regressive tax: it places a disproportionate burden on the worse-off. There are ways of avoiding that problem, however, including subsidies on a means-tested basis.

When we consider the possibilities for moral constraint, there is reason for both pessimism and optimism. On the positive side, some people who could afford to purchase ever-bigger homes, newer fancier automobiles, and state-of-the-art personal computers do *not* do so. They seem to have grasped the economists notion that sometimes "satisficing" is better than optimizing—or, more accurately, that "local" optimization is not always optimal from a "global" point of view that takes the full range of values, including spontaneity, into account.

Similarly, some people (in fact at this point a majority of people in the United States) seem to exercise sufficient restraint not to become morbidly obese, even though high-calorie, heavily marketed fast-food is cheap enough that they could easily do so. (This is *not* to say that obesity is always or even in most cases a matter of lack of restraint, but only that many people have the potential to become overweight but don't and that at least for some of them this is at least in part a matter of self-restraint.)

On the negative side, the economist Robert Frank and others have shown that, at least in contemporary American culture, there is a strong current of "luxury fever"—a dissatisfaction with good-quality possessions and an endless quest for "higher quality."[18] It is possible that this propensity will become focused on biomedical enhancements rather than (or even worse, in addition to) the currently highest quality material possessions. Frank's point is that the unbridled quest for "higher quality," in a society in which mass marketing is potent, results in less well-being, not more, for some people. Loss of spontaneity is only one way in which well-being may decrease; I have explored others in discussing the bad consequences of the failure to appreciate existing goods.

At the beginning of this chapter I noted that some of the most vociferous critics of enhancement say that they are not concerned primarily with the bad consequences of the pursuit of enhancements. Instead, they say they are worried about what the very pursuit of enhancements says about our character. It turns out, however, that at least some character concerns, in their most cogent form, are in fact worries about consequences. We have just seen that the most illuminating way to understand rhetoric about mastery, perfectionism, and "gratitude" may be as a set of predictions about the results of the widespread availability of biomedical enhancements: a worsening of tendencies to fail to appreciate existing goods, to engage in inappropriate self-manipulation/objectification and to leave too little room in one's life for spontaneity as one comes to exist almost exclusively in the goal-pursuing mode.

It is important to emphasize this consequentialist dimension of character concerns for two reasons. First, it makes clear that *the strength of these considerations against enhancement depends on the reliability of the predictions involved and the ability to supply empirical evidence to support them.* Second, *even if the predictions can be empirically supported, they are, like other predictions, conditional: they assume that certain background conditions are satisfied.* They do not assert that X will occur no matter what, but rather that X will occur if conditions C1, C2...CN persist.

Because they are conditional predictions, the outcomes they predict can be avoided—if we can alter the background conditions. For example, the large-scale excessive pursuit of biomedical enhancements, like the large-scale excessive pursuit of better cars, depends upon the items in question being affordable to great numbers of people. As I have already noted, that condition will be undercut if costs are sufficiently increased.

Adapting to enhancement

I now want to suggest that in trying to assess the validity of character concerns about biomedical enhancement we should consider the diachronic dimension. Here the analogy with obesity is instructive. Whether or not there is an "obesity epidemic" in the United States, it is true that more people have higher body mass indexes nowadays and that when one's body index becomes high enough, some health risks increase. It also seems likely that this development has to do with the emergence of a radically new situation in human affairs: the almost instant availability, twenty-four hours a day, of cheap, high-caloric food to a population that does far less physical labor than preceding generations.

There is no reason to assume that we will be able to adapt instantaneously to this novel situation. Perhaps some time is needed to learn to cope with this situation and perhaps some people, depending upon their socio-economic and educational status and the array of skills and resources that correlate with these indicators, will learn more quickly than others. A similar claim might be made regarding the availability of cheap distilled spirits in England 250 years ago: people accustomed to drinking large quantities of weak beer were suddenly able to buy gin, and the social skill of drinking hard liquor in moderation was not acquired instantly or uniformly across classes. (For a vivid depiction of the devastating consequences of the availability of cheap gin in England, see Hogarth's "Gin Street.")

I am not making a prediction that "the problem of obesity" will subside because more people will learn how to control the ratio between calories ingested and calories burned; nor am I predicting that people will learn how to resist "biomedical enhancement fever" (if there ever comes to be an epidemic of it). My point is simply this: those who raise character concerns about biomedical enhancement that turn out to be predictions about the consequences of the widespread availability of these technologies ought to recognize that such predictions are not only conditional but may also be time-bounded, depending upon how we adapt to new possibilities. They also ought to acknowledge that such predictions are not self-evident truths, but empirical hypotheses requiring empirical support.

The burden of empirically based argument that would have to be borne to translate predictions about the effects of the widespread availability of biomedical enhancements into sound arguments against the enhancement enterprise is a heavy one. So far, no critic of enhancement has begun to shoulder it. In Chapter Six, I will consider the question of where the burden of argument lies under conditions in which our knowledge of the likely outcomes of pursuing the enhancement project is limited.

Inauthenticity

One of the more interesting character concerns is that the widespread use of biomedical enhancements—and especially mood enhancing drugs—will result in inauthenticity. Talk about authenticity is heady stuff, but notoriously obscure. In this section, I attempt to sort out the more significant concerns and evaluate them. It will prove useful to distinguish and consider in turn worries about inauthentic selves (or lives), inauthentic relationships, and inauthentic (or pseudo-) excellences.

Inauthentic selves

Carl Elliot has suggested that if one gets a "new personality" from taking a mood-enhancing drug like Prozac, one's life will be inauthentic, because in some important sense the new self will not be one's own.[19] To begin to understand this seemingly paradoxical claim, we need to settle on a working definition of authenticity, as applied to selves or human lives. Suppose we begin—tentatively and provisionally—with the idea that an individual lives authentically if and only if she is "true to herself."

In a valuable article in which he challenges Elliot's suggestion, David DeGrazia spells out being true to oneself in terms of acting in ways that are consistent with one's identity.[20] "Identity" here means (roughly) one's reflective, settled conception of one's self, an understanding of who one is that embodies one's most stable, highest priority values. There are many different conceptions of identity and their suitability may vary depending upon the context. In discussing the risk that the use of mood enhancement drugs may undercut the conditions for living authentically, DeGrazia's understanding of authenticity seems to me to be a promising starting point.

I wish to offer a friendly amendment to it, however. For this context, our conception of authenticity should rule out cases in which one's conception of oneself—one's identity in DeGrazia's sense—is grounded in delusions or grossly false beliefs or determined in significant ways by "scripts" that have been foisted on one by others through techniques akin to brainwashing or through coercion. The point is that for a being capable of rationally forming beliefs about how to live and to be, living in accordance with delusional or merely parroted values is living inauthentically.

For our purposes, it will not be necessary to work this idea out in any detail. Instead, we can simply add to DeGrazia's conception of authenticity as identity an *epistemic proviso*—a qualification to rule out conceptions of the self that are either grossly delusional or palpably slavish. The basic idea is that authenticity, in the sense worth caring about, is more than simple congruity between one's behavior and *some* conception of what sort of person one aspires to be. Even perfect harmony between one's life and one's self-conception would not be authenticity, so far as authenticity is a virtue, if one's self-conception were either grounded in grossly false beliefs or in a "script" that one has internalized without critical reflection. One might go further and say that a life lived in conformity with a self-conception that is merely a parroted script is not authentic because such a self-conception is itself inauthentic. From now on when I refer to authenticity as living in accordance with one's identity, I will mean identity as qualified by an appropriate epistemic proviso.

DeGrazia argues that even if using Prozac produced such a profound change as to make sense of the notion of having a new personality, the result would be an authentic life, if the choice to use the drug was a voluntary expression of one's identity, that is, if it was in accordance with and undertaken to further one's stable, highest priority values about how to live and what kind of person to be. I agree that some rather profound changes in personality are compatible with authenticity on any reasonable understanding of what authenticity is, including DeGrazia's. Yet I also believe that we need to qualify this conclusion by taking the epistemic proviso into account. If the conception of oneself that one was trying to realize through taking Prozac was based on grossly delusional beliefs or was merely a script foisted on one by others, then the resulting "new personality" might be inauthentic, in fact, less authentic than one's personality before taking the drug. If the availability of powerful pharmaceutical mood enhancement drugs made it easier for people to live their lives according to conceptions of the self that are based on deeply delusional belief systems or to follow parroted scripts, then this enhancement technology could worsen whatever risks of living inauthentically we now face.

Notice again the familiar shift: we start out with a worry, or in some cases a bold assertion, that a biomedical enhancement is an *instance* of inauthenticity; but then on closer inspection we see what is really at issue is an empirical claim, a prediction that the technology *will worsen the risks of living inauthentically that we already face.* What we need, but do not presently have, in order to convert this concern into a significant practical conclusion, is empirical evidence to support the proposition that the added risk is great enough—relative to the benefits of the enhancement—to warrant either an attempt to prevent the further development of mood-enhancing drugs, or some policy that aims to constrain their availability or regulate their use.

The unduly protean self

I have already noted one respect in which the use of powerful mood-enhancing or personality-changing drugs may be more problematic from the standpoint of authenticity than DeGrazia thinks: under conditions in which some people's self-conception is itself "inauthentic," either because it is delusional or merely parroted, equipping them with technologies that enable them to make themselves conform to such a self-conception may make their lives less, rather than more, authentic. But there is another problem: being authentic, on DeGrazia's view, means living in accordance with one's self-conception, but for this conception of authenticity to make sense, there must be a core self that is relatively stable. For talk of being true to oneself to have traction, there must be a self to be true to. This point does not depend upon the assumption that there is an unchanging psychological core. It may be that all we need to make sense of the idea of being true to oneself is significant continuities and connections among a series of psychological states, to use Parfit's terminology.[21] Perhaps part of what concerns some of us about the prospect of extremely powerful enhancement technologies, especially if they include drugs that produce profound psychological changes, is that they might make us too malleable, too protean. Alexandre Erler argues that living authentically means, *inter alia*, showing proper regard for one's present self and that such regard places moral constraints on the use of mood or personality-enhancing drugs beyond those which DeGrazia's account allows us to recognize.[22] In other words, on Erler's view, being "true to oneself" means more than acting in conformity with one's self-conception; it means exhibiting a degree of loyalty to one's present self. Because one's self-conception is a blend of description and ideal—partly a view about how one is and

but self growth is key & amazing!

partly about how one ought to be—there can be a discrepancy between what is required by a proper loyalty to one's present self and what one needs to do to realize one's self-conception. Erler thinks that in some cases being authentic means refraining from altering one's present characteristics, even if doing so would be an improvement and a better realization of one's self-conception.

Erler's view is subtle and interesting. I cannot do it justice here. I would like to point out, however, that neither the concern about excessive malleability that I have raised nor Erler's worry about failing to show a proper regard for one's present self need be framed in terms of risks to the authenticity. There are other, more tangible and less controversial moral concepts that are directly applicable.

Consider first the problem of excessive malleability or lack of continuity. Even if he maintains his identity in some sense, an individual who altered his most morally significant psychological characteristics too abruptly or too frequently could go wrong in several ways. He could disrupt the legitimate expectations of others and he could destroy valuable relationships that depend upon greater continuity than his protean life possesses. Whether or not such a protean life can be authentic, it is morally defective in other ways.

A similar point might be made about proper self-regard. We might think of this as a matter of authenticity, but we might instead understand it as an application of an idea already encountered: that of proper appreciation for existing good. Even if one could become better through using some biomedical enhancement, in some circumstances utilizing the enhancement may show a lack of appreciation for the value of one's present self. Sometimes showing a proper appreciation of an existing good is best achieved by preserving that good, even while recognizing its limitations. It would certainly be inappropriate to be constantly entertaining ideas about how a friend or lover or family member could be improved, much less to be urging them toward perpetual improvement. A person who did this could plausibly be accused of not adequately appreciating the other individual as he or she is. A similar attitude of relentless improvability toward oneself might be equally inappropriate, whether it was a threat to authenticity or not. Perhaps this, too, is a concern that is being gestured at, though in a not very illuminating way, by rhetoric about the pursuit of enhancement being "perfectionism."

The familiar pattern repeats: what at first appear to be damningly tight links between the pursuit of enhancements and vices or distorted values turn out, on careful inspection, to be highly speculative, complex contingent connections whose existence and robustness depends upon a complex set of variables, some of which may be within our control. Whether the use of mood or personality-altering drugs for enhancement will result in inauthenticity or in overly protean lives will depend upon how malleable the human psyche turns out to be, upon how costly these interventions are, upon whether people will be able to see that much of what we rightly value depends upon a significant degree of psychological continuity and connectedness and to act effectively on this realization.

Inauthentic relationships: the case of "love drugs"

In a provocative, empirically well-informed, and insightful paper, Julian Savulescu and Anders Sandberg examine the ethics of using "love drugs" to sustain human pair-bonding.[23] I want to build on this discussion in order to explore the question of whether, or under what circumstances, biomedical enhancements are a threat to authentic relationships.

Savulescu and Sandberg begin by identifying a problem and then suggest that chemical enhancement might contribute to its solution. The problem is that the biochemical basis of human pair-bonding decays after the reproductive years, while contemporary social conditions, when taken along with evolved, fairly generalized sexual attraction, create the risk that couples will become estranged from one another. Some people may wish to reduce this risk, for the sake of preserving what they regard as a valuable relationship and an important part of a good life, and for the sake of their children.

Some rather dramatic research indicates that mammal pair-bonding is highly malleable in response to biochemical changes. One species of vole is "monogamous," another not. In the laboratory, both by insertion of genes and by administration of the chemicals oxytocin and vasopressin, "monogamous" voles have been converted to being not monogamous and vice versa.[24] The same chemicals and genes are present in primates, including human beings, and there is reason to believe their physiological effects are similar.[25]

Suppose it becomes possible (and safe) to take a drug that will increase the probability that one will remain sexually faithful. Suppose that there is mounting evidence that one significant factor in the breakdown of marriages or other long-term relationships is that there is an evolved rather general (relatively nondiscriminating) sexual response in humans and that the drug works by dampening this generalized sexual response or by making it more amenable to rational control. Alternatively, suppose that the drug works by heightening (or sustaining) one's sexual response toward one's mate.

There is some evidence that men are, on average, somewhat more prone to sexual infidelity in marriage than women, though the difference may be diminishing.[26] Some evolutionary psychologists believe that this is an evolved biological feature of males; some social psychologists explain it as an artifact of the prevalence of patriarchal cultures in which men have the power to be unfaithful with relative impunity and to impose severe costs on female infidelity. Either way, a male who highly values sustaining a long-term relationship with one woman, and his partner, should be worried—and worried enough to consider whether there are ways to reduce the risk.

Savulescu and Sandberg ask whether it would be morally permissible to use this enhancement technology. They conclude that it could be. They point out that human beings have long used low-tech pair-bonding enhancements (alcohol, flowers, provocative clothing, poetry, beach vacations without the kids, second honeymoons, etc.). I pointed out to these authors another nonbiomedical pair-bonding preservation strategy: in some states people are able to opt for a "fault" rather than "no fault" marriage contract, which increases the costs of divorce and thereby adds incentives for staying married.

This last example is clearly an instance of what I have called rational self-manipulation. Presumably the people who avail themselves of the "fault" marriage option do so because they value stable marriages, while recognizing that under contemporary conditions, the combination of economic and social incentives and "natural" biochemical attractions may not be sufficient. They fear they will yield to temptation and they take a deliberate step to subject themselves to additional costs that they hope will enable them to resist it. Presumably, opting for "fault" marriage or taking other nonbiomedical approaches to helping ensure marital stability can be morally permissible. If so, why wouldn't taking a drug be morally permissible as well?

Earlier in this chapter I argued that rational self-manipulation, including self-binding, is not in itself morally impermissible. If that is the case, then perhaps we should conclude that chemical enhancement of pair-bonding is morally unproblematic as well. Under the factual assumptions set out above, using a "love drug" would be a case of trying to counteract a morally problematic feature of our evolved biological make-up or a morally problematic cultural tendency. It would not be the pursuit of perfection or a quest for mastery. The motivation for using the "love" drug would be admirable, not tainted, so using it wouldn't betray bad character or distorted values.

There is a further question, however: Would a relationship that is sustained in part by the use of such drugs be authentic? The answer to that question depends upon exactly what relationship one is referring to. More specifically, one might well wonder whether a relationship that is chemically sustained would be love. That is an ill-framed question, for two reasons. First, without further clarification about what is meant by "love" here, it is impossible to answer. There are different cultural conceptions of love and there may be different—and contested—conceptions of love within a given culture. Once we specify which of these we are talking about, we can ask whether it is even relevant to the question at hand.[27] For example, if one is operating with certain conceptions of romantic love, then many people who value stable marriages or long-term relationships (perhaps especially if they belong to non-Western cultures) may be quite unconcerned about whether chemical enhancements are compatible with romantic love. They may think, quite reasonably, that romantic love is not essential to a good marriage. Second, neither Savulescu nor anyone else, so far as I know, is claiming that the administration of oxytocin or vasopressin or any other drug can *create* a long-term relationship that is loving under any reasonable conception of what love is. The claim is much more modest: that the use of these drugs can increase the probability that a couple will stay together by counteracting biological and/or cultural factors that can undermine their commitment to one another. That claim is compatible with there being a number of different kinds of commitment and a plurality of kinds of valuable long-term relationships. The chemical strategy assumes, quite reasonably, that there are other factors besides love that influence the prospects for a long-lasting union, but so does the "fault" marriage strategy.

In considering the issue of authenticity, it is important to avoid the mistake of thinking that the proposal is to *introduce* a chemical factor into the relationship. The point is that our biochemistry *already* plays a role in sustaining relationships. If the fact that biochemistry plays a role in human pair-bonding (and always has) doesn't render relationships inauthentic, then it cannot be the case that the deliberate administration of the same drugs itself robs the relationship of authenticity.

except that it's an "administration" not a natural reaction.

That could occur only if the drugs were so powerful as to override voluntariness. If the drug *compelled* one to continue in the relationship, then at least on some conceptions of love, the relationship would not be an authentic loving relationship. We have now slipped into the fantasy world of the Valley of the Dolls (or even more grimly, that of the serial killer Jeffrey Dahmer, who injected battery acid into the skulls of his victims in a rather unscientific attempt to make them his "love slaves"). But we are supposed to be talking about love drugs, not love zombie fantasies.

The idea of enhancement "love drugs," on its more plausible interpretation, is that they increase the probability of fidelity by doing something to counteract the effects of cultural or biological risk factors, not that they determine behavior. It is worth noting, however, that on the contrary assumption, namely, that vasopressin and oxytocin *compel* attraction, there is a worry about authenticity, but it arises with respect to "natural," not biomedically enhanced, pair-bonding. If we are pawns of our sexual biochemistry, then the idea that our choice of partners is an expression of our identity is an illusion. Authenticity might *require* using biomedical interventions to avoid attractions that are not expressions of our identity or to stimulate or sustain attractions that are in accordance with it.

hmmm

Some might reply that the "natural" biochemical basis of pair-bonding is compatible with authenticity, but that the "artificial" support renders pair-bonding inauthentic because it is "artificial." Authentic relationships, they might say, are those that are based on the biochemistry we are "given" by nature. Authentic relationships are based on our nature and taking "love drugs" interferes with that nature.

PERIOD :)

This line of thinking is so defective that it is hard to know where to begin in criticizing it. In the next chapter (Human Nature and the Natural) I explore it in detail. Here I will only make two points. First, as John Stuart Mill pointed out long ago, in one sense it is impossible to interfere with Nature (unless one can perform miracles); in another, we interfere with Nature all the time and often it is a good thing.[28] In the first sense of "Nature," nature is simply the totality of the natural world, subject to whatever natural laws there are. In the second sense, Nature is opposed to human agency; in this sense, we speak of letting Nature take its course as opposed to our acting. But in the second sense, it is not only morally permissible but also morally obligatory to interfere with Nature in many cases—for example, to administer insulin to diabetics. If, as many evolutionary psychologists contend, human males are especially prone to sexual infidelity as a result of their evolved characteristics, and if what evolution has produced in this case is an obstacle to achieving what we rightly value, then we *ought* to "interfere with Nature." If what we value highly as a result of informed reflection is a monogamous relationship — to use DeGrazia's phrase, if that is part of our morally defensible identity—then using drugs to counteract evolved tendencies that pose obstacles to our acting in accordance with our "identity" is not acting inauthentically. On the contrary, simply allowing our relationships to be undermined by a combination of biological and social risk factors, when we could effectively and safely counteract them by chemical or other means, would be failing to be true to ourselves.

Of course, a number of complex questions about the ethics of using "love drugs" remain to be explored. It is important to understand, however, that the topic is not a new one. It has been the stuff of fables, plays, and novels for centuries (think of the romantic comedies, such as *The Tempest*, whose plots turn around misdirected administrations of "love drugs," or tragedies, such as *Tristan and Isolde*, where the ingestion of a "love drug" is unwitting). I make no pretense of exploring this rich domain in this volume. My point is only that there is nothing wrong or inauthentic *per se* with enhancing one's capacity to sustain a valuable relationship through the use of drugs or other biomedical interventions.

The risks of rational self-manipulation

Any form of rational self-manipulation, whether biomedical or "traditional," carries risks. I have already noted one of them: one may fail to treat oneself respectfully, acting as if one were merely an object rather than a being with the capacity for autonomy. I have also explained how treating oneself in this way could result in the loss of spontaneity or of the continuity needed for commitments and stable relationships. There are other risks as well. One might, for good reason, change one's mind about the relationship, but find it impossible, or too costly, to extricate oneself from it because of the effectiveness of one's self-binding or other rational self-manipulation strategy. The incentives or other causal influences created through rational self-manipulation might prove so powerful as to render one's commitment to the relationship less than voluntary. In some cases, the rational self-manipulation technique itself might change the character of the relationship for the worse. (For example, entering into a "fault" marriage, or setting up a prenuptial financial agreement, might prompt suspicions that would undermine trust.) In addition, effective and relatively easy rational self-manipulation techniques might tempt some people to rely on them too much, shirking some of the hard but necessary work of sustaining a relationship.

These are all significant risks. They are not peculiar to *biomedical* rational self-manipulation for purposes of enhancement, however. How serious they are will vary, depending upon the type of rational self-manipulation employed, the psychology of the individuals involved, and other circumstances. In a particular case, the risks might be unacceptably high. But that does not show that rational self-manipulation in general or when it utilizes biomedical enhancement is incompatible with authentic lives or authentic relationships or is otherwise morally suspect.

Inauthentic virtues

There is one more character concern worth considering. Some might object to the very idea that biotechnologies could produce moral enhancements, if this means making us more virtuous. They would regard the states of character that are produced by such interventions as inauthentic—as pseudo-virtues. Real virtues, they would contend, are not created in that way.

In what way? The point cannot be that a virtue isn't genuine unless it came to be solely through the efforts of the individual himself, through direct exercises of his will, so to speak. On that criterion, no one would ever possess any authentic virtues. The development of virtues never comes about solely through the individual's exercise of will. It comes about through the operation of a number of factors, including the deployment by his parents and other mentors of an array of techniques.

For example, parents use moral education techniques of various kinds, including punishment and exposure of the child to the influence of persons of good moral behavior, which help to form and to sustain the child's character. Such traditional techniques do not operate solely through the child's will or choice—they are typically instigated without the child's consent and include coercive restrictions on her liberty. Yet the results they help to achieve are authentic virtues. If anything, an improvement in character that results from one's reflective, identity-affirming choice to take a drug that enables one to develop one's capacity for empathy or moral imagination would appear to be *more* authentic than an improvement that results from the exercise of parental power over an unconsenting child.

When an adult, for the sake of improving or sustaining his character, chooses to subject himself to certain influences that will then operate independently of his will, as in self-binding or forms of rational self-manipulation involving positive incentives, whatever virtues he has do not thereby become inauthentic. Being virtuous does not come about solely through exercises of the will. Similarly, sustaining virtue also frequently—perhaps always—requires causal influences that are not directly answerable to the will. Perhaps the most crucial of these influences are social: a person who lives in a society in which many people are virtuous or at least in which being virtuous is not generally a disadvantage has a better chance of continuing to be virtuous, other things being equal. If a person lives in social circumstances that are conducive to the preservation of a virtue, then his continuing to possess it may be *less* attributable to the exercise of his will than it would be if he had helped to sustain it by a biotechnological intervention. But this would not lead us to conclude that his socially supported virtue is not genuine virtue. So, *a fortiori*, the fact that biomedical interventions, once put in play, operate independently of the will cannot render the virtues they help to create or to sustain inauthentic.

If a person somehow succeeded in attaining or sustaining virtue solely through her own efforts, she would be especially commendable. But from that it doesn't follow that relying on others or on causal influences to which one deliberately subjects oneself as in rational self-manipulation is morally wrong. On the contrary, choosing to rely solely on one's resolve would be morally wrong if it put one at unacceptable risk for acting immorally or for losing the virtues one possesses. Under these circumstances, steadfast refusal to avail oneself of moral enhancements, biochemical or otherwise, would be a vice—the vice of hubris. The path of argument in this chapter has been long and winding. I hope to have given concern about the implications of biomedical enhancement for character a more balanced hearing than the critics of enhancement have done. At the very least, I believe that I have sorted out various character concerns more clearly than they have. My chief conclusion is simple: legitimate worries about character are not conclusive reasons against the enhancement enterprise, much less against biomedical enhancements across the board; at best they are considerations to be taken into account in the responsible use of enhancements.

Notes

1. As per Michael Sandel (2007), *The Case Against Perfection: Ethics in the Age of Genetic Engineering* (Harvard University Press), pp. 99–100.
2. See ibid.
3. See Stephen Pinker (2003), *The Blank Slate: The Modern Denial of Human Nature* (Penguin Press Science), p. 222.
4. Thomas Douglas (2008), "Moral Enhancement," *Journal of Applied Philosophy* 25(3): 228–245. Halley Faust (2008), "Should we select for genetic moral enhancement? A thought experiment using the MoralKinder (MK+)," *Theoretical Medicine and Bioethics* 29(6): 397–416; Mark Walker, "Genetic Virtue" (unpublished manuscript, available at http://ieet.org/index.php/IEET/more/4741).
5. For a discussion of the selection of "pro-social" traits, see Thomas Douglas and Katrien Devolder, "Wide Procreative Beneficence: Beyond Individualism in Reproductive Selection" (unpublished manuscript).
6. G. Jones (2008), "Are Smarter Groups More Cooperative? Evidence From Prisoner's Dilemma Experiments, 1959–2003," *Journal of Behavior and Organization,* 68(3–4): 489–497.
7. A. Tversky and D. Kahneman (1981), "Framing Decisions and the Psychology of Choice," *Science* 211(4481): 453–458; Linda Babcock *et al.* (1995), "Biased Judgments of Fairness in Bargaining," *American Economic Review* 85(5): 1337–1343; C. Goldin and C. Rouse (2000), "Orchestrating Impartiality: The Impact of "Blind" Auditions on Female Musicians," *American Economic Review* 90(4): 715–741.
8. Sandel 2007, supra note 1, pp. 82–92.
9. Ibid., p. 96: "I am suggesting . . . that the moral stakes in the enhancement debate are not fully captured by the familiar categories of autonomy and

rights, on the one hand, and the calculation of costs and benefits, on the other."

10. Michael Sandel (2004), "The Case Against Perfection: What's Wrong With Designer Children, Bionic Athletes, and Genetic Engineering?" *The Atlantic Monthly* 292(3): 51–62.
11. See Roger Scruton (2001), *The Meaning of Conservatism*, 3rd edn., St. Augustine's; Russell Kirk (2001), *The Conservative Mind: From Burke to Eliot*, 7th edn. (Regnery Publishing).
12. G.A. Cohen, "Rescuing the Truth In Conservatism" (unpublished paper).
13. Giuseppe di Lampedusa (1960), *The Leopard*, translated from the Italian by Archibald Colquhoun. (New York: Pantheon Books).
14. See Martin Heidegger (1998), "The Question Concerning Technology," in *Basic Writings*, D.F. Krell, (ed.) (HarperCollins).
15. I owe this point to Thomas Douglas.
16. I am indebted to Tom Hurka for making this point clear to me.
17. Ingmar Persson and Julian Savulescu (2008), "The Perils of Cognitive Enhancement and the Urgent Imperative to Enhance the Moral Character of Humanity," *Journal of Applied Philosophy* 25(3): 162–177.
18. Robert Frank (2001), *Luxury Fever*, new edn. (Princeton University Press).
19. Carl Elliot (1998), "The Tyranny of Happiness," in *Enhancing Human Traits. Ethical and Social Implications*, Erik Parens (ed.) (Washington, DC. Georgetown University Press), pp. 177–188.
20. David DeGrazia (2000), "Prozac, Enhancement and Self-Creation," *Hastings Center Report* 30(2): 34–40.
21. See Derek Parfit (1986), *Reasons and Persons* (Oxford University Press), p. 286.
22. Alexandre Erler, dissertation manuscript.
23. Julian Savulescu and Anders Sandberg (2008), "Neuroenhancement of Love and Marriage: The Chemicals Between Us," *Neuroethics*, 1(1): 33–44.
24. Miranda Lim *et al.* (2004), "Enhanced Partner Preference in a Promiscuous Species by Manipulating the Expression of a Single Gene," *Nature* 429 (6993): 754–757.
25. See e.g. Bales KL, Mason WA, Catana C, *et al.* (2007), "Neural correlates of pair-bonding in a monogamous primate." *Brain Research* 1184: 245–253.
26. D.C. Atkins, D.H. Baucom, and N.S. Jacobson (2001), "Understanding infidelity: Correlates in a national random sample," *Journal of Family Psychology* 15(4): 735–749; R.J. Brand, C.M. Markey, A. Mills, and S.D. Hodges (2007), "Sex differences in self-reported infidelity and its correlates," *Sex Roles* 57: 101–109.
27. My discussion here has benefited from an interesting unpublished paper on biomedical enhancement of pair-bonding by Jonathan Sides.
28. John Stuart Mill (1904), "On nature," in *Nature, The Utility of Religion and Theism* (Watts & Co.).

CHAPTER FOUR

Human Nature and the Natural

Critics of enhancement voice two concerns about the impact of enhancements on human nature. The first is that enhancement may alter or even destroy human nature.[1] The second is that if enhancement alters or destroys human nature, this will undercut our ability to ascertain the good, because, for us, the good is determined by our nature.[2] The first concern assumes that altering or destroying human nature would be a bad thing. The second concern assumes that human nature provides a perspective without which we cannot make coherent, defensible judgments about what is good.

I aim to show that neither of these concerns is cogent. I will argue (1) that there is nothing wrong, *per se*, with altering human nature, because, on plausible understandings of what human nature is, it contains bad as well as good characteristics and because there is no reason to believe that in every case efforts to eliminate some of the bad characteristics would pose an unacceptable risk to the good ones. I will also argue (2) that if the eventual cumulative result of a series of biomedical enhancements were to "destroy" human nature by replacing us with beings that were "posthuman," that would not be wrong in itself and might in fact be a good thing. In addition, I will show (3) that altering human nature need not result in the loss of our ability to make judgments about the good, because we possess a conception of the good by which we can and do evaluate human nature. This means that we have an evaluative perspective that is to some extent independent of our nature. Finally, I will argue (4) that appeals to human nature tend to obscure rather than illuminate the debate over the ethics of enhancement, and can be eliminated in favor of more cogent considerations.

In this chapter I distinguish several conceptions of human nature, articulate five different roles that appeals to human nature can play in Ethics, and explain their implications for the enhancement debate. Next I examine one appeal to human nature that has been especially prominent in the enhancement debate, the view that reflection on our nature can supply substantive moral rules, including a prohibition on enhancements that would alter or destroy our nature. I then argue that this latter view, which I call normative essentialism, is irreparably flawed. Finally I probe the idea of human nature as a whole, a set of complex interdependencies. I argue that the worry that biomedical enhancements might disrupt complex dependencies can be more fruitfully expressed without recourse to the concept of human nature.

Scientific knowledge, as opposed to a prior speculation or folk wisdom

Those who adamantly oppose enhancement insist that a sound ethical approach to enhancement must include an understanding of our proper relationship to nature and especially to our own nature. Since their critique of enhancement depends crucially on appeals to nature and human nature, one would think that these anti-enhancement writers would take seriously the issue of how claims about nature and human nature are to be justified. Surprisingly, they do not. They seem to be oblivious to how controversial claims about human nature often are—and how mistaken even the best thinkers of the past have been about them. Instead of relying on the best knowledge we have of nature—modern biology informed by Darwinian evolutionary theory—they ground their ethical critique of enhancement in *a priori* speculation. Even worse, as I shall show, their speculations are directly at odds with our scientific knowledge.

Of course, some people may base their understanding of nature on faith or religious revelation, rather than on science. Interestingly, the critics of enhancement whose work I examine in this volume do not take this line. They *claim* to be raising objections to enhancement based on appeals to nature or human nature that are accessible to secular discourse. But if one is examining the ethics of enhancement within the framework of secular discourse, then whatever one says about the relationship between enhancement and nature or human nature ought to be informed by our best scientific understanding of nature. By claiming to frame the issues within the confines of secular discourse but at the same time ignoring the relevance of science for claims about nature and human nature, these critics put themselves in an untenable situation. In this chapter and more fully in the next, I argue that it matters a great deal as to whether one frames issues concerning the ethics of enhancement in terms of a scientific understanding of nature and human nature, or rather on the basis of *a priori* speculation that is inconsistent with the central features of evolutionary biology.

Different roles for the concept of human nature in ethics

At least since Aristotle, the dominant philosophical conception of human nature is that of a set of characteristics that are common to all humans and that distinguish humans from other kinds of beings. If one adds the assumption that there are natural kinds, then these characteristics are thought of as essential, rather than merely contingent. From this it follows that if any of these characteristics disappeared, we would no longer be human beings.

There are less philosophically sophisticated conceptions of human nature as well, both secular and theological. According to what might be called folk (or colloquial) conceptions, human nature consists of a set of dispositions that all (or at least most) humans have and that shape behavior across a wide range of human activities, regardless of cultural context, throughout human history. There is much disagreement about which characteristics manifested by human beings fit this description. It has been said that human beings are selfish by nature, or that they tend to have biases against members of "outgroups," that it is human nature to seek the transcendent, to love one's offspring and to be prepared to make sacrifices for them, to be prone to fall foolishly in love, to rationalize about one's failings, to be sociable, to be capable of knowing the laws of reason, to be able to make moral judgments, etc. Some contemporary evolutionary biologists and neuroscientists would say that if the concept of human nature has any value it is as shorthand for those "hard-wired"[3] characteristics that most humans now have as a result of their common evolutionary development.[4] Contemporary social scientists who are impressed by the role of culture and by the interaction of biology with culture would say that human nature includes both biological "hard-wiring" and certain universal, or at least very widely prevalent, culture-based dispositions. Common to all of these conceptions of human nature is the idea that if something is part of human nature it is recalcitrant to alteration by acculturation, education, or indoctrination, and stable across a wide variety of environments. This is true even of conceptions of human nature that include a cultural element, because those culture-based dispositions that are said to be part of human nature are thought to be inculcated at a very early age and rendered highly stable by social institutions and practices. Neither folk, nor biological, nor biological–cultural conceptions of human nature need include the assumption that everything that is part of human nature is unique to humans, as the example of sociability indicates (some nonhuman animals are social). Further, unlike traditional metaphysical conceptions of human nature as essences, none of these conceptions of human nature requires strict universality: they require only that the traits in question are widely distributed enough for appeal to them to play a major role in explaining human behavior.

Side-stepping the debate about competing conceptions of human nature

Nothing I say in this chapter or in the remainder of the volume requires me to adjudicate the complex debate about whether a concept of human nature plays an important role in biology or social psychology or if so which particular conception of human nature is apt.[5] I do want to suggest, however, that to make the discussion that follows more understandable, we can begin with the following highly general characterization of the concept of human nature. This concept can be spelled out in a number of different conceptions.

Human nature is a set of characteristics (1) that (at least) most individuals who are uncontroversially regarded as mature human beings have; (2) that are recalcitrant to being expunged or significantly altered by education, training, and indoctrination; and (3) that play a significant role in explanations of widespread human behavior and in explanations of differences between humans and other animals.

This characterization has several advantages, for our purposes here: it avoids the problematic pre-Darwinian idea of fixed essences, it does not require strict universality of traits included in human nature, and it is general enough to cover a wide range of more specific folk, biological, cultural–biological, and religious conceptions of human nature. It also makes clear the relevance of scientific knowledge. To know which characteristics (if any) meet conditions (1), (2), and (3) in the definition, we have to look to a scientific investigation of the way we are.

Human nature and goodness

Conceptions of human nature usually do not restrict human nature to *good* characteristics. Folk conceptions typically include the idea that human nature has a dark side. Religious conceptions often hold that human nature includes sinfulness. Biological conceptions employ the concept of fitness, not goodness, but they are compatible with judgments about the goodness or badness or those traits that are said to be part of human nature. For example, if certain dispositions are now part of our nature because they evolved during what evolutionary theorists call the ancestral evolutionary environment, they may be not only maladaptive in our current, quite different environment, but also bad from the standpoint of our moral values. Conceptions of human nature that include cultural elements distinguish between what makes a cultural group sustainable and what is just or good for individuals or minorities within it, and also acknowledge the possibility that culture-based traits that at one time were beneficial may become deleterious, as can happen with biological traits.

Could biomedical interventions alter or destroy human nature?

On any of these quite different conceptions of human nature, altering human nature would presumably require at least this much: large-scale changes to one or more of the characteristics that have been common to all or most normal human beings. The qualifier "large-scale" is intended to indicate that if such changes occurred only in some but not most human beings, we would probably say that *they* had become something other than human, rather than that human nature had changed.[6] A neutral term for the different sorts of beings that might replace human beings as the cumulative result of many biomedical enhancements over time is "posthumans."

On the general concept of human nature set out above, could a series of enhancements, undertaken on a large scale, eventually culminate in the emergence of *posthumans*—beings sufficiently different from us that it would make sense to regard them as other than human beings, as having a nature different from that of human nature? Given that we are only beginning to create biotechnologies that could be used for enhancement, it is difficult to say. There is one reason *not* to assume a negative answer to the question, however: in the past, evolution has produced new kinds of beings, including human beings, and enhancement biotechnologies of the future may be able to produce similar changes, if not on their own, then in combination with evolutionary changes.

Once we give up the pre-Darwinian idea that species have fixed essences and think of the traits that we associate with human nature as historical products that persist for a time and are then replaced with new ones, we cannot rule out the possibility that similar changes could occur again, by deliberate human design or through a combination of "natural" evolution and deliberate design. Nor can we rule out the possibility that at some point the cumulative effects of such changes might make it reasonable to conclude that a new kind of being, a being with a different nature from our own, had emerged. If this occurred, posthumans might coexist with humans (as Neanderthals did for a time with our ancestors). Moreover, we cannot assume that coexistence would persist; the emergence of posthumans might eventually result in the extinction of human beings.

Before we are swept away by such giddy speculations, however, it is important to see that mere increases in strength, longevity, cognitive or emotional functioning, or resistance to disease—the sorts of enhancements now most discussed—would not result in posthumans. Colloquial conceptions of human nature, as well as the biologist's concept of *Homo sapiens*, are presumably capacious enough to accommodate a good many such changes, so at this point predictions that enhancement will usher in a posthuman future may be premature. To produce a new conceptual–explanatory scheme in which the concept of a human being was replaced by that of a posthuman, the changes that enhancements brought would have to be widespread and would also have to produce significant qualitative differences, not merely higher levels of existing traits. For example, merely enhancing the human immune system, increasing average IQ by twenty points, and extending life by 50 years would not produce posthumans. These sorts of changes would not call for anything as radical as the recognition of a new hominid species.

Nevertheless, as difficult as it may be for us to imagine what sort of changes would require the recognition of a new species, we cannot dismiss the possibility that they could come about through the cumulative effects of increasingly powerful biomedical enhancements over a long period of time. In principle, biomedical enhancements appear to be capable of transformations as significant as those that evolution has produced in the hominid lineage in the past.

Appeals to human nature in Ethics

To begin to evaluate concerns about the impact of enhancement on human nature, it will prove useful to distinguish different roles that the idea of human nature (HN) has played in Ethics. Five different roles may be distinguished: (1) HN as a condition of practical rationality and hence of moral agency, (2) HN as a feasibility constraint on morality, (3) HN as a constraint on the good for humans, (4) HN as a source of substantive moral rules, and (5) HN as a whole that exhibits *extreme connectedness*—a complex set of densely interdependent characteristics—that is likely to be seriously damaged by efforts to improve it. Each of these roles will be explained and in each case the implications for the enhancement debate will be explored. The discussion that follows makes no pretence to completeness; that would be hubristic, given the many different ways in which the term "human nature" has been used. It should suffice to show, however, that objections to enhancement based on appeals to human nature are either otiose or ineffectual.

HN as including a precondition for moral agency

Practical rationality, understood as the capacity to recognize and act on reasons or, in Kantian terms, to be motivated to act by the belief that one ought to do something, has often been regarded as an important constituent of human nature. On some views, including Kant's, to destroy our capacity for practical rationality would be perhaps the deepest wrong. But no one advocating the moral permissibility of enhancements is suggesting that the destruction of our capacity for practical rationality would be an enhancement. So, the only relevance of this first sort appeal to human nature in ethics is simply to warn us to beware of one especially bad possible unintended consequence of efforts to enhance, namely, the inadvertent destruction or impairment of our capacity for practical rationality. Saying that we should take care not to damage our capacity for practical rationality in the pursuit of enhancements sheds very limited light, however, on the question of whether we ought to undertake any particular enhancement that is likely to be proposed. Moreover, the concern about damaging our practical rationality can be expressed without recourse to the concept of human nature.

HN as a feasibility constraint on morality

Some moral philosophers, including Hume and contemporary practitioners of "neuroethics"—the study of the implications of neuroscience for Ethics—emphasize that a properly realistic understanding of morality must take into account the cognitive and motivational limitations of human beings (the "hard-wiring" we happen to have as a result of evolution). If, for example, by virtue of our evolved biological make-up, we have a limited capacity to act altruistically toward strangers, then a plausible account of our moral obligations to others must take this into account. "Ought" implies "can" and what we can do is limited by our evolved biology.

There is an obvious reason why this sort of appeal to human nature sheds scant light on the ethics of enhancement: included among the enhancements with respect to which we seek moral guidance are those that would involve the removal or relaxing of the very sorts of limitations that Hume and neuroethicists emphasize. Suppose it becomes possible, for example, to administer drugs that increase our ability to empathize with strangers and hence to be motivated to act altruistically toward them.[7] What had been a limitation on the human capacity for altruism would to that extent be relaxed.

Regardless of whether a given limitation thought to be part of human nature is alterable or not, this second sort of appeal to human nature, like the first, can do little work in the ethics of enhancement. On the one hand, if a current motivational or cognitive limitation *can* be removed or relaxed by some biomedical technique, then the question is whether it would be a good idea, all things considered, to remove or relax it. The fact that until now we have been subject to this limitation tells us nothing about whether we should continue to be so. This point is especially clear and obvious if we think of human nature in the way evolutionary biologists do: the most we can say about any characteristic that is part of human nature is that it, or some characteristic to which it is tied in the processes of human biological development, *was* adaptive at some point in the development of our species. We cannot assume that it is still adaptive at present, much less that it will be adaptive in the future or that it is inextricably tied to something that is or will be adaptive. On the other hand, if a particular limitation is unalterable, then there is no issue of whether altering it is permissible and the idea of that it is a part of human nature adds nothing to the claim that it is unalterable. In either case, the appeal to human nature as a set of limitations on human motivation and cognition and hence on morality does not advance our understanding of the ethics of enhancement; nor does it lend support to the thesis that it is wrong *per se* to change human nature.[8]

What is more, the very technologies that have prompted the enhancement debate also call into question the usefulness of the concept of human nature, insofar as it includes the idea of unalterability. These technologies challenge the idea that we have a fixed core of characteristics.

HN as a constraint on the good for us.

In one plausible interpretation, Aristotle held that a being's nature determines its good, but only in a rather minimal sense: by constituting a constraint on what can count as a good life for that kind of being. According to this view, if human beings are by nature rational, then the good life for human beings, whatever else it is like, must include significant scope for the exercise of reason. Similarly, if human beings are by nature sociable, then the good life for them must include ample scope for social interactions.

This third sort of appeal to human nature, like the preceding two, is of meager value in wrestling with the ethics of enhancement. It neither forbids nor condones enhancements that would alter our nature, because it merely says that in seeking the good, we should remember that a being's nature constrains its good. By itself, this reminder is silent on the question of whether we should continue to live under the constraint that our nature imposes. Consider this analogy: if we are limited to a particular canvas, we can only create a painting that fits within its boundaries and we should take that into account in deciding what to paint—*on it*. But if we have the option of using *a different* canvas, then

there will be other possibilities (and other constraints, as well). Recognizing that a given canvas limits the artistic good we can achieve does not
imply that we should refrain from changing canvasses; nor does it imply
that we *should* change canvasses. But it does raise the question of whether
there might be reasons for using a different canvas, if we can. We might
come to realize that if we changed our nature in a certain way, we would
become capable of goods that are not available to us but that would be
worth pursuing.

Perhaps some aspects of our nature constrain our good in unfortunate
ways. To revert to an earlier example: our limited altruism may cut us off
from forms of sociability that would greatly improve the quality of our
lives. If such were the case, the question would be whether this sort of
enhancement could be safely achieved and whether it would be good, all
things considered. As I have already noted, in attempting to answer this
question we would have to take the risk of unforeseen bad consequences
very seriously.[9]

Knowing whether an intervention would be a good thing all things
considered is a daunting task; but it is not made easier by recourse to the
notion of human nature. Nor can an appeal to the concept of human
nature help us decide whether, in the face of such uncertainties, it would
be best to adopt some version of a Precautionary Principle or some other
set of cautionary maxims that would function to counterbalance tendencies to underestimate risks in the pursuit of benefits. (In Chapter 7,
I explore the idea of cautionary maxims or heuristics in considerable
detail.)

Alternatively, suppose that we see no reason to try to "paint on a new
canvas." Suppose also that we agree that sociability, rationality, compas-
sion, etc., are aspects of our nature which, given our resolution to seek
the good within the constraints of our nature, we should do nothing to
imperil. What follows about whether we should undertake this or that
biomedical intervention for the sake of enhancement? Not much, for the
simple reason that the plausibility of saying that any such characteristic is
part of our nature depends upon characterizing it in a very abstract
fashion. Consider sociability, for example. Sociability is a good candidate for being something that all normal humans have the capacity for,
and which is deeply ingrained if not innate; in that sense one might say
that sociability is part of human nature. But a moment's attention to
cultural diversity indicates that sociability can take many forms. There is

a dilemma, then. Either one characterizes the features of human nature that are to constrain our pursuit of the good very abstractly, in order to make more plausible the claim that they are in fact features of human nature and not merely characteristics that some humans have, in which case they can provide few limitations on the sorts of enhancements we might opt for. Or, one characterizes them in more determinate ways, so that the notion that they are to be preserved can significantly constrain our options regarding enhancement, but at the price of rendering implausible the claim that they are really features of human nature, rather than characteristics that some humans have.

Nevertheless, it is conceivable that a biomedical enhancement of some human capacity would damage some human capacity we rightly value, for example, our capacity for empathizing with others. If this damage occurred, then our capacity to achieve the good, to live well, might be seriously compromised, but not because our capacity for empathy is part of our nature; rather, because the capacity for empathy is either itself an important component of our good or instrumental for other goods, or both.[10]

The argument thus far can now be summarized. Beyond being an unnecessary circumlocution for an admonition to avoid unwittingly destroying capacities upon which our good depends, the idea that human nature is a constraint on the good for us cannot supply much content for an ethics of enhancement. Nor can it provide an argument for the claim that we should not change our nature, because it only tells us that if we have a certain nature, that should be taken into account when we try to determine what our good is, not that we should persist with that nature and the constraints on goodness that it entails. Finally, to the extent that the case against improving human nature rests on the assumption of extreme connectedness, it requires scientific backing. One cannot merely assume that connectedness is so thoroughgoing as to rule out any attempts at improvement.

HN as a source of substantive moral rules: normative essentialism

Some of the harshest critics of enhancement, including Leon Kass and the President's Council on Bioethics, which he chaired for a time, embrace what might be called *normative essentialism*: they believe it is possible to derive substantive moral rules from reflection on human nature. More specifically, they believe it is possible to derive moral rules that include a prohibition on enhancement and on reproductive cloning as well. For example, the Council's *Report on Human Cloning and Human Dignity* solemnly declares that "human reproduction is sexual" (meaning that it involves the combining of genetic material from a male and a female) and then proceeds as if this is a strong and even a conclusive reason against cloning, which is a type of asexual reproduction.[11] It is important to understand that the Council's claim is *not* simply the descriptive statement that so far human reproduction has been sexual, that is, has involved the uniting of a sperm and an egg. That statement, though true (virgin births aside), would by itself give us no reason whatsoever to oppose asexual reproduction, including cloning. (That would be like answering the question "Should we go to Paris?" by saying "We haven't gone to Paris in the past.") The Council clearly advances the claim that human reproduction is sexual as a *moral* claim, not as a description of our practice so far. Its claim is that sexual reproduction is the only form of reproduction that is natural *in the sense of being fitting for human beings or in keeping with the dignity that their nature bestows.* So, on the Council's view, any attempt at enhancement that involved cloning would be impermissible. For the Council, the connection between the "unnaturalness" of cloning and of enhancement is clear: The Council report, *Beyond Therapy*, sees cloning as opening the door to a "new eugenics" that would involve not only "selecting out" undesirable traits, but also engineering desirable ones, and not necessarily just those falling in the normal range.[12] The Council also makes the prediction, without even gesturing toward evidence to support it, that the use of biomedical enhancement techniques involving the design of human embryos would convert procreation (a "natural" activity for human beings) into "manufacturing" (a mode of producing human offspring that is contrary to the "natural" way of doing so).[13]

The Council's claim is not simply that the engineering of human embryos would produce bad results, but that it would alter our nature, "distorting" natural (and therefore good) human relationships. According to this view, human nature comprises not only certain capacities that individual human beings have, but also certain kinds of relationships among human beings. The fear is that some kinds of relationships that might emerge from the widespread use of biomedical enhancements would be "unnatural," that is, contrary to human nature and damaging to it. In addition, it is assumed that our good is inextricably tied to our nature in a very determinate way: altering our nature would undermine our good. This assumption overlooks the obvious possibility that altering some characteristics that are part of our nature might increase our opportunities for good.

The crucial point is that the adjective "human" in "human reproduction is sexual" is being used by the Council as a normative, not a purely descriptive term. The clear implication is that asexual reproduction and hence cloning is debasing, demeaning, unnatural, or even perverse—in a word, less than human. Similarly, the Council states that in procreation "a man and woman give themselves in love to each other, setting their projects aside in order to do just that."[14] Taken as a descriptive claim, this is surely false as a generalization, unless one simply equates love with sex (which the Council would never do), because human procreation sometimes has nothing to do with love. So, taken at face value as a descriptive claim about what procreation is, it has the bizarre implication that many human beings are not produced by procreation. (How *are* they produced, then? Imagine this headline: "President's Council determines that millions of people are not produced by procreation!") In addition, as a descriptive claim, it rules out by definitional fiat the possibility of same-sex partners procreating. So if biomedical technology eventually made it possible to create an individual by combining DNA from partners who were of the same sex, this would not be human procreation, according to the Council's stipulative definition of human procreation as sexual (in the sense of involving the combining of DNA from a male and a female). As a normative claim, it implies that if same-sex partners could procreate this would be *inhuman* or *less than human* and that the same is true when men and women procreate without the procreative act being an act of love.

Notice that even if it is true that procreation that involves love is *better* (other things being equal) than procreation that does not, it does not follow that procreation which is not an act of love between a man and woman is *impermissible,* less than human, or incompatible with the fundamental dignity of humanity. Ironically, while sternly criticizing enhancement as the quest for perfection, the President's Council pins one of its chief arguments against enhancement on an unspoken assumption that anything that departs from what they assume to be the

best sort of human procreative activity is wholly unacceptable, demeaning, and subhuman.

The Council's appeal to normative essentialism is perhaps clearest in
its criticism of cloning, but it is also implicit in the critique of enhancement in the report *Beyond Therapy*. This is not surprising, since, as
I have already noted, the Council explicitly links cloning to enhancement, viewing it as the doorway to a "new eugenics" that would "alter
the nature" of human procreation by converting "begetting" into
"manufacturing."[15] In its discussion of the possibility of genetic interventions in human embryos to enhance normal human characteristics,
the Council states that "The salient fact about human procreation in its
natural context is that children are not *made* but *begotten*. By this we
mean that children are the issue of our love, not the product of our
wills."[16] As I have already noted, taken as a descriptive generalization,
this last statement is clearly false: in many cases children are not the issue
of love (they are often the result of careless sex and sometimes of rape)
and in some cases they are the product of human willing, as when people
deliberately try to conceive an heir or to produce another child to take
care of them in old age or to help them with subsistence agricultural
work. If the Commission's point is simply that the practice of genetically
engineering our offspring would involve a new connection between
willing and procreating—namely, the choosing of a child's genotype—
that is certainly true, but adding that this would be a departure from "the
natural context" does nothing to show that it would be wrong. Moreover, "the natural context" here is just a misleading way of referring to
the status quo—the way things have been done up until now. To say
that the way things have been done is the natural way is unilluminating
at best and false at worst, since in many cases the way things have been
done is simply a result of cultural practices. Moreover, not all sexual
reproduction is "natural," even in the sense of being the way humans
have done things traditionally. Procreation using IVF (*in vitro* fertilization) is sexual reproduction in the Council's sense: it involves the
combining of DNA from a male and a female (in the laboratory), but
it is a very recent development.

The Council also claims (again without offering any data) that "we"
find repulsive the idea of 70-year-olds having children and suggests that
this reaction of repugnance indicates that such an extension of the
normal period of human reproductive activity would be contrary to

what is "naturally human," with the clear implication that this counts against such a development.[17] Whether or not reproduction at the age of seventy is a bad idea would depend on how vigorous 70-year-olds are like, how long they are likely to live, etc.—and all of that could be quite different in an era of biomedical enhancements.

The key point, however, is that the fact that some people, even most people, find something repulsive does not show that it is unnatural in any way, much less that it is unnatural in a normative sense that implies that it is wrong to do it that way. If people a generation or two ago were told that girls were beginning to menstruate at the age of eleven or twelve, they might find this "unnatural" and even repugnant, but that would presumably be a result of the fact that they lived in a society in which nutrition was so poor that female development usually only allowed the onset of menstruation to occur much later. Whether beginning to menstruate at the age of eleven or twelve (as opposed to eighteen or twenty in the eighteenth century) is a good thing is a different question altogether.

The Council does not rely entirely on the implication that genetically designing children would be "unnatural" in its condemnation of enhancement. Instead, it goes on to suggest that genetically designing embryos is either equivalent to or will lead to the replacement of the "natural" activity of procreating with a process of manufacturing children. The description of current procreation as "natural" in this claim, however, does no argumentative work: the issue is whether genetically designing embryos is or is likely to lead to parents regarding their offspring as manufactured items. Reference to human nature or the natural can be eliminated without loss.

The Council's attempt to link genetic enhancement with "manufacturing" is ambiguous. The claim could be that if the practice of genetically designing embryos for purposes of enhancement becomes common, then there will be a deleterious change in the attitude of parents toward children: parents will come to regard their children as artifacts, manufactured items, not as persons in their own right. This is an empirical prediction, but neither the Council nor anyone else who makes it offers evidence to support it. One place to begin to look for evidence would be to do careful studies of the attitudes of parents toward children that have been born as a result of genetic selection of embryos. The Council does not do this, however, or even suggest that it should be done. Until we have evidence that selecting or designing embryos does in fact produce such a profound change in the character of parenting, it is hard to know what to make of the stern declaration about manufacturing. At the very least, it seems rather premature to rule out all instances of selection or design simply because the widespread use of these techniques *might* undermine good parenting in some instances. Without empirical evidence, the "might" here merely indicates that the outcome the Council fears is consistent with what we know about human psychology; it doesn't mean that the outcome is likely. Proceeding on the assumption that one should avoid activities that might produce harmful results is a recipe for paralysis, not prudence.

There is another interpretation of the claim that parents who genetically design embryos in an effort to enhance the capacities of their children are engaging in "manufacturing" rather than procreating, one that makes it a conceptual claim about every instance of genetic designing of embryos, rather than an empirical prediction about the effects of a widespread practice. On this interpretation, to attempt to influence one's child's characteristics by inserting genes into the embryo from which she will develop just *is* to treat her as a manufactured item.

That is a staggeringly implausible claim. People might insert genes in embryos for any number of reasons, some of them quite admirable and fully compatible with recognizing that the child that will be born will be a person, not a mere thing. This would be the case if the goal were to increase the probability that the child will have a temperament of the sort that is generally conducive to happiness or to achieve some enhancement of normal cognitive functioning, or to enhance the normal human immune response in order to provide protection against emerging pandemics, or to enhance the body's capacity for thermal regulation in order to mitigate the ill-effects of global warming. To say that to design an embryo for purposes of enhancement *is* to engage in manufacturing rather than procreating only makes sense if one is willing to disregard commonsense (and moral probity) and declare that anyone who engages in this mode of enhancement has bad motives or doesn't recognize the difference between a widget and a child. We have already seen, in Chapter Three, just how unconvincing and how sleazy this mode of attack is.

It should now be evident that the problem with normative essentialism is not merely that it disguises normative claims as descriptive claims. If that were the only problem, it could be solved by reformulating the claims in a way that makes their normativity obvious. There is a deeper flaw. Normative essentialist claims confuse two quite different kinds of moral judgments, and fail to provide justifications for either: judgments about what is best for human beings and judgments about what is compatible with human beings' fundamental moral status or dignity. It is one thing to claim that a certain way of procreating is best, or even that other ways of procreating are in some way defective. Such judgments are controversial enough and normative essentialists typically do not take up the burden of providing plausible justifications for them. It is even more problematic to assert that anything other than this particular way of procreating is *less than human, incompatible with human dignity—even subhuman.*

The history of prejudice and persecution is replete with normative essentialist claims: homosexuality is unnatural, marriages between the races are unnatural, social equality for inferior and superior types of humans (e.g., Aryans and non-Aryans, Nietzschean "higher-types" and "lower-types") is unnatural, demeaning (to the superior), etc. That alone should make one suspicious of normative essentialist claims and prompt an insistence that they be backed up with evidence or argument. What sort of backing do Kass and the President's Council provide for normative essentialist claims like "human reproduction is sexual" or that "in procreation a man and a woman give themselves to each other in love"?

Most who are skeptical of such claims have focused on Kass *et al.*'s appeal to "the wisdom of repugnance." Kass *et al.* have acknowledged the simple but powerful point that feelings of repugnance can be not just unreliable, but counter-reliable (as when a racist feels repugnance upon seeing a White person and a Black person kissing). But they have not begun to take up the burden of articulating a moral epistemology that would enable us to distinguish between those feelings of repugnance that reveal moral truth and those that do not. And they have certainly not articulated a normative account of human nature that would either explain which feelings of repugnance are veridical or make the appeal to such feelings unnecessary for determining what is permitted and what is not.

The history of Ethics indicates that such an account is unlikely to be forthcoming. Reflection on the concept of human nature can provide some constraints on the good for humans, but it is not a source of substantive moral rules that could decide controversial moral issues, at least not rules prohibiting homosexuality, mixed marriages, or asexual reproduction.

The normative essentialist faces a destructive dilemma. If the concept of human nature from which controversial substantive moral rules (prohibiting asexual reproduction or enhancement, or procreation by same sex partners, etc.) are supposed to be derived is itself normatively rich enough to ground those rules, then that highly normative concept of human nature will itself be equally controversial and no argumentative leverage will be gained. But if the concept of human nature the normative essentialist invokes is thin enough to be plausible to those who do not already accept the substantive moral rules that are supposed to be derived from it, then it will be too thin to ground those rules. In either case, the appeal to human nature does not help us resolve enhancement issues.

It would be unfair to Kass *et al.* to let the matter rest there, however. They might concede that feelings of repugnance and reflection on the concept of human nature are insufficient to ground the very strong and determinate moral prohibitions on cloning and enhancement they advance. Instead, they might recast their view roughly as follows.

A good human life is one in which there are certain relationships—between parent and child, between men and women, among siblings, between older and younger generations. The goods that flow from these relationships are deeply interdependent; altering any of them not only entails a loss of the good that it involves, but also threatens to undermine other goods. Sexual reproduction (i.e., reproduction involving a genetic contribution from a male and a female) is one important aspect of the good life for human beings; it is valuable in its own right but is also connected, through various interdependencies, to other important human goods. So, abandoning sexual reproduction in favor of reproduction by cloning or abandoning traditional parenting in favor of parenting that includes the designing of embryos would imperil the good life for humans.

This version of the Council's message avoids normative essentialism: it does not attempt to resolve moral controversies by deriving substantive moral rules from reflection on the concept of human nature and it seems to dispense with unsupported and question-begging pronouncements about what is fitting for human beings or in keeping with their dignity. Instead, it appeals to the idea of a good life and to the interdependency of goods within it. Call this the Good Life Argument, to distinguish it from normative essentialism.

The first thing to notice about this new argument is that it is not an attempt to show that cloning or enhancement or anything else is wrong *because it would alter or destroy human nature.* Thus it avoids the problems of normative essentialism.

This gain comes at an exorbitant price, however. Proponents of the Good Life Argument must bear an enormous burden of empirical evidence to make plausible their sweeping claims about the relevant causal interdependencies. Once again we encounter the unsupported assumption of extreme connectedness. They have to show, in effect, that the good life is a seamless web, that severing one fiber is likely to result in the whole thing unraveling. Empirical evidence, not armchair speculation, must be marshaled to show that the various aspects of the good human life are so thoroughly interdependent. In particular, there must be credible evidence for the claim that if asexual reproduction or procreation by same sex partners or the genetic enhancement of children become common, this will undermine various relationships that the argument assumes to be of great value.

Notice that it will not do to state, as the Report does, that cloning or the designing of children will "confound" relationships between generations. If "confound" is an evaluative term, meaning roughly "distort" or "derange," then this claim presupposes precisely what is at issue, namely, that the fitting, proper, true or natural relationship between individuals is precisely the one that has obtained until now, before the possibility of the biomedical intervention in question; and the argument therefore collapses back into naked normative essentialism. If, instead, the term "confound" is shorthand for the assertion that certain biomedical interventions will in fact disrupt certain causal dependencies, then this is an empirical claim that needs evidence.[18]

The facts of cross-cultural diversity suggest that this daunting burden of empirical evidence is not likely to be borne. Some societies now recognize same-sex marriages and homosexuality and all include reproduction that has more to do with sex or economics than love. (To borrow the Council's sonorous biblical phrasing: many people are not "begotten.") Yet it appears that good human lives are possible within such societies, even for those who depart from the Council's standards of "naturalness," and this suggests either that the behavior in question is not bad or that if it is bad, the goodness in human life is much more independent of it and more resilient than the seamless web metaphor implies.

Further, Kass *et al.* must argue, not assume, that the forms of human relationships they believe are endangered by cloning or enhancement are not only goods (objectively speaking, not merely things *they* happen to value), but also goods of such overwhelming value that they can never be reasonably compromised for other goods. Simply to declare that certain kinds of relationships or activities (male–female parenting, sexual reproduction, parenting that does not involve genetic intervention in embryos, etc.) are so valuable that they must never be imperiled for the sake of any other good, is to beg the question in an argumentative context in which their opponents do not agree with the Council's particular perfectionist theory of the good. Here we encounter again the irony noted earlier: those trying to make a case against perfection do so from the standpoint of a very dubious perfectionism.

My argument thus far can now be summarized. The type of argument against enhancement (and cloning) that the Council advances either relies on the concept of human nature and is an unpersuasive normative essentialist argument, an attempt to derive substantive and controversial moral rules from the concept of human nature; or instead presupposes a very controversial, perfectionist theory of the good and an unarticulated and ambitious empirical social science theory to support very strong claims about the causal interdependence of the elements of a good human life, neither of which its proponents have begun to articulate, much less defend.

Human Nature as a Complex Whole

The assumption of extreme connectedness

Sometimes the term "nature" or "the natural" is used to convey the idea of a complex whole, a dense web of harmonious interdependencies, as when those concerned about the effects of human activity on the environment speak of the disruption of Nature. In the enhancement context, the worry is that if we change any part of human nature, even an undesirable part, we endanger the good parts as well.

Some enhancement critics, and in particular Fukuyma and President Bush's Council on Bioethics, have argued for a ban on enhancements as the proper response to the risk that in trying to make ourselves better we might destroy something of great value. Fukuyama, says that "... we want to protect the full range of our complex, evolved natures against attempts at self-modification."[19] Presumably, Fukayama would agree with commonsense that our natures include some items that are less than optimal and some that are bad. So he appears to be assuming that "we" don't want to change anything because it is too risky, given the interdependence of the good and the bad.

Given that some enhancements might bring great benefits, this extreme response to the problem of risk would make sense only if the extreme connectedness assumption were valid and if there were no less drastic effective strategies for reducing risk. As I shall argue in Chapter Six, there are such strategies. The simple point I wish to make here, however, is that one is likely to exaggerate the risk of bad unintended consequences—and hence be less receptive to a consideration of risk reduction strategies short of a total ban on enhancements—if one assumes extreme connectedness. To assume extreme connectedness is to make a sweeping generalization about the facts of human biology, namely, that it is characterized by such a thoroughgoing interdependency of functions that it is always too risky to try to modify any part of it. Critics of enhancement who implicitly assume extreme connectedness do so from the armchair; they do not even begin to make the case that this sweeping hypothesis is supported by biological science.

In Chapters Five and Six, I will argue that evolutionary biology, rather than supporting the extreme connectedness assumption, gives us reasons to doubt it. Here I only want to note that even if there were good empirical evidence for a claim about connectedness that was strong enough to ground an absolute prohibition on efforts to enhance, the result would not be a sound argument from human nature to an anti-enhancement conclusion but rather the abandonment of any role for an appeal to human nature in the argument. What matters is whether proposed enhancements are likely to produce bad unintended consequences because of our ignorance of interdependencies that support what is valuable; whether the things that are interdependent are parts of our nature is irrelevant. Once again, the appeal to human nature is eliminable without loss.

Focusing on connectedness, not human nature

In brief, if the appeal to human nature is simply shorthand for an appeal to the fragility of wholeness—to the dangers of meddling with complex interdependencies—it is shorthand we can do without. Moreover, relying on this kind of shorthand is not only unnecessary, it is pernicious to the extent that it encourages the delusion that reflection on human nature can yield substantive moral rules capable of resolving controversies about enhancement. Having to grapple with the ambiguity of the notion of human nature and to resolve long-standing disputes about what is and is not included in human nature simply distracts attention from the issue of connectedness. Chapters Five and Six explore the role that assumptions about extreme connectedness play in anti-enhancement analogies and arguments, and subject those analogies to scrutiny in the light of evolutionary biology.

Human Nature and the Ability to Judge What is Good

Once we appreciate the implausibility of normative essentialism, we are in a better position to evaluate the charge that enhancement could, by altering or destroying human nature, undermine our ability to make judgments about the good. The idea here is that human nature provides a standard for the good in the following sense: to know whether something is good (for us) we need to know whether it conforms to or is consistent with or "fits" our nature. I have already suggested one reason to reject the claim that if we alter our nature we will lose the capacity to make judgments about the good. I have argued that the role that the appeal to our nature plays in making judgments about the good is that of providing a constraint on what can be good for us, *so long as that is our nature*. Therefore, altering our nature need not result in the inability to judge what the good is. An altered nature could simply supply new constraints.

There is a second, more important reason to reject the claim that an alteration in our nature would rob us of the ability to make judgments about the good: we already make what appear to be perfectly sound evaluative judgments about human nature, judgments that can supply reasons for altering that nature. For, as I have already observed, human nature is typically thought to include bad as well as good characteristics. It is said that to be human is to be selfish, to be inclined to excessive partiality, or to be sinful, for example. The idea that human nature is a mixed bag is perhaps most credible in the case of evolutionary conceptions of human nature: there is no reason to assume that all of the human traits that have evolved are good.

Whether or not the claim that some aspects of human nature are bad is true, there seems to be nothing incoherent about it. But if that is so, then it appears that we have a standard of goodness that is somewhat independent of our concept of human nature. In principle, then, there seems to be nothing wrong with the idea of changing those parts of our nature that are bad, if this can be done without imperiling the good parts. To assume otherwise is to beg the question at hand, to assume, rather than to argue, that changing human nature is itself a wrong. Further, we can give reasons—just the sort of reasons that we use to support judgments about the good in other cases—for why it would be good, other things being equal, to alter some of the more unsavory traits which, on some views, are part of human nature. For example, suppose, as some evolutionary biologists claim, that it is part of human nature—a widespread trait due to our evolutionary past—that we have a bias toward negative evaluations of those we regard as alien, as "not one of us." Perhaps if this propensity were reduced, there would be fewer wars and a reduction of the miseries that wars bring. The reasons we would have for changing this putative aspect of human nature are familiar reasons, reasons having to do with what is bad for us, with what tends to undercut our well-being. So to that extent, we already have an evaluative perspective that is independent of our nature and changing some aspect of our nature need not result in the inability to make well-grounded judgments about the good.

Nor is there reason to assume that if such changes were made, we would no longer be able to make coherent judgments about the good. Even if our capacity to make evaluative judgments is in some way dependent upon our nature, it does not follow that it is dependent on each and every aspect of our nature.

It might be replied that the idea of human nature is nonetheless needed to flesh out an adequate conception of *our* well-being, to distinguish it from the well-being of other animals. For example, it could be argued that our well-being requires that we have the capacity for complex and self-conscious forms of sociability, for a degree of autonomy (the capacity to lead a life, not just to live), etc.

All of that is no doubt true, but it can be said without invoking the idea of human nature, where this means a set of characteristics that is universal in all humans and unique to them. Presumably if there are intelligent extraterrestrials, then the capacity for complex, self-conscious forms of sociability and for autonomy will be important for their well-being, too, even if they were not human beings. If we say that certain capacities that we believe (perhaps wrongly) are peculiar to human nature are important for our well-being, all the normative work is being done by the idea that they are important for well-being, not by the claim that they are part of our nature.

Consider one last interpretation of the claim that our capacity to judge the good depends upon human nature and hence could be imperiled by efforts to alter human nature through the application of biomedical technologies. Suppose that the capacity to make judgments about goodness is part of human nature, where human nature is understood, not as the problematic metaphysical notion of essence, but simply as a bundle of properties that most normal, mature members of our biological species have and that is not possessed (*in toto*) by any other creatures on earth. Depending upon how robustly we construe the capacity for judging goodness, it may be plausible to say that this capacity is part of human nature in this metaphysically lean sense. If a biomedical intervention had the unintended consequence of destroying the capacity for judging goodness, then it would follow trivially that *this* alteration of human nature undercut our capacity for judging goodness. But it would not follow that *any* alteration of our nature would undercut that capacity. So, even if it is true that the capacity for judging goodness is part of human nature, it does not follow that by altering human nature we undercut our ability to judge goodness. Here, as elsewhere, we can eliminate the appeal to human nature and focus instead on the commonsensical admonition to try to avoid enhancement efforts that may have unintended bad consequences.

Conclusion

I have argued for the following theses. (1) The fact that an enhancement would alter or destroy human nature is in itself not a reason to forgo the enhancement. Setting aside the difficulties of determining which of our characteristics are part of human nature (and in which sense of that ambiguous term), the question is whether we have good reason to try to change a particular characteristic. The answer to that question will depend upon a number of factors, including whether the characteristic is undesirable on balance and whether in attempting to change it we would put at unacceptable risk things we rightly value. Whether it is part of our nature is irrelevant, unless by stipulative definition we say that what is part of our nature is impossible to change, in which case the appeal to human nature is nothing more than an otiose admonition not to try to do what cannot be done. (2) Reasonable worries about enhancement that are sometimes expressed in the language of human nature—such as the concern about unintended consequences due to unnoticed interdependencies between what we wish to change and what we wish to preserve—can be more clearly expressed without appealing to human nature. Because appeals to human nature in this context are not only unnecessary, but also run the risk of degenerating into the errors of normative essentialism, they are best avoided. (3) It is not the case that in altering human nature we would *thereby* undermine our ability to make judgments about the good. We already possess standards of evaluation that are independent of our nature in the sense that we can and do make coherent judgments about the defective aspects of human nature, and if those defects were remedied this need not affect our ability to judge what is good.

My critique of appeals to human nature and the natural in this chapter has been directed against contemporary bioethicists who invoke these notions in opposition to enhancement. Their deployment of the notions of human nature and the natural has been shown to be naïve and superficial in the extreme: they proceed as if they were unaware of how problematic talk about human nature is, as if statements about human nature need not take evolutionary biology into account, as if the history of Ethics vindicated, rather than exploded, normative essentialist attempts to derive substantive normative conclusions from the concept of human nature, and as if the long history of oppressing people by branding their relationships as "unnatural" or less than human had never occurred.

Notes

1. For some relevant literature, see Harold W. Baillie and Timothy K. Casey, eds. (2004), *Is human nature obsolete? Genetics, bioengineering, and the future of the human condition* (Cambridge, MA: MIT Press); Leon Kass (2000),

140   *Human Nature and the Natural*

"The Wisdom of Repugnance," in *The Human Cloning Debate,* 2nd edn., Glenn McGee (ed.), pp. 68–106. (Berkeley, CA: Berkeley Hills Books); and Erik Parens (ed.) (1998), *Enhancing Human Traits: Ethical and Social Implications* (Washington, DC: Georgetown University Press).

2. Two prominent examples include Jürgen Habermas (2003), *The Future of Human Nature* (Cambridge: Polity), and Francis Fukuyama (2002), *Our Post-Human Future: Consequences of the Biotechnology Revolution* (New York, NY: Ferrar, Straus & Giroux).

3. "Hard-wired" here does not mean deterministic. Rather, it is used to convey the idea that the dispositions in question are recalcitrant to modification by training, education, and acculturation (hence the adjective "hard"), and also that their existence is more innate than learned.

4. See for example Stephen Pinker, *The Blank Slate: The Modern Denial of Human Nature,* 2003, Penguin Press Science.

5. For a discussion, see E. Machery (2008), "A Plea for Human Nature," *Philosophical Psychology* 21: 321–330.

6. Norman Daniels (2009), "Can anyone really be talking about ethically modifying human nature?" in *Enhancement of Human Beings,* Julian Savulescu and Nick Bostrom (eds.) (Oxford: Oxford University Press).

7. For example, serotonin is thought to play a role in suppressing aggression in normal individuals. J. Haller, E. Mikics, J. Halasz, and M. Toth (2005). "Mechanisms differentiating normal from abnormal aggression: Glucocoricoids and serotonin," *European Journal of Pharmacology* 526(1–3): 89–100. The relationship between serotonin levels and aggression does not appear to be simple, however. See V. O'Keane, E. Moloney, H. O'Neill, A. O'Connor, C. Smith, and T Dinan (1992), "Blunted Prolactin Responses to D-fenfluramine in Sociopathy. Evidence for Subsensitivity of Central Serotonergic Function," *The British Journal of Psychiatry* 160: 643–646. Oxytocin is a hormone that facilitates birth and breastfeeding in humans and other mammals. It also appears to facilitate maternal care and pair-bonding in some nonhuman animals. T.R. Insel and R.D. Fernal (2004), "How the Brain Processes Social Information: Searching for the Social Brain," *Annual Review of Neuroscience* 27: 697–722.

8. Some critics of enhancement, including Michael Sandel and Erik Parens, contend that enhancement is objectionable precisely because it involves the removal of limitations on what human beings can do, because they believe that there are irreplaceable goods that depend upon our having limitations. See Erik Parens (1995), "The Goodness of Fragility: On the Prospect of Genetic Technologies Aimed at the Enhancement of Human Capacities," *Kennedy Institute of Ethics Journal* 5(2): 141–53, and Michael Sandel (2004), "The Case Against Perfection," *The Atlantic Monthly* 293(3): 50–62. For a systematic critique of this view, see Allen Buchanan (2009), "Human Development and Human Enhancement," *Kennedy Institute Journal of Ethics* 18: 1–34.

9. Notice that it would be a mistake to assume that an enhancement that altered an individual's nature—that made her no longer a human—would result in the loss of that individual's identity. Personal identity could be preserved through such a transformation, regardless of whether one assumes that personal identity requires only continuity of psychological states or that plus the persistence of the body. Such a change would result in the loss of the individual's identity only if it were true that persons are essentially human.

10. I am grateful to Tom Douglas for this point.

11. President's Council on Bioethics (2002) *Human Cloning and Human Dignity: An Ethical Inquiry* (Washington, DC: National Bioethics Advisory Commission).

12. President's Council on Bioethics (2002), *Beyond Therapy*, (Washington, DC: National Bioethics Advisory Commission), p. 70. Here the Council says that cloning and eugenic interventions might "alter the very nature" of human procreation.

13. President's Council on Bioethics 2002, supra note 11, pp. 99–101, 104–107.

14. Ibid., p. 99.

15. President's Council on Bioethics 2002, *Beyond Therapy*, supra note 12, p. 70.

16. Ibid., p. 70.

17. Ibid., p. 287.

18. Perhaps the claim that cloning would "confound" relationships among generations is a clumsy shorthand for the empirical psychological prediction that if reproduction by cloning were pervasive people would be confused and disturbed in their thinking about the relationships among generations. The Council provides no evidence for this prediction and no indication of how serious or pervasive the alleged psychological distress would be. Nor do they address the fact that there is evidence that people can adjust, rather rapidly, to new reproductive technologies, for example, IVF. Despite some initial speculation that "test-tube babies" would be regarded as freaks, most people seem to have taken IVF in stride.

19. Fukuyama 2002, supra note 2, p. 172.

CHAPTER FIVE

Conservatism and Enhancement

The strongest denunciations of enhancement come from those who are plausibly categorized as Conservatives. Kass, Fukuyama, and Sandel are prime examples. The objections of these Conservatives do not seem cogent because they appear to appeal, uncritically, to what is natural, as if the natural were always good, or to a supposedly widespread repugnance to enhancement, without any account of how we are to distinguish morally significant repugnance from mere distaste or prejudice. Above all, the complaints of contemporary Conservative bioethicists about enhancement lack philosophical depth: they seem ungrounded in any coherent, systematic, carefully worked out moral and political view. And yet the suspicion lingers that there just may be something to the worries that Conservative bioethicists have about enhancement and that they are, in some important sense, genuinely *Conservative* worries. It seems reasonable, therefore, to explore the best resources of the rich Conservative tradition, in order to see whether Conservative bioethicists' concerns about enhancement can be expressed more adequately. That is what I do in this chapter.

I will draw on what might be called the mainstream Burkean tradition of Conservative thought, try to determine its bearing on enhancement, and ask whether it supplies good reasons for refraining from the enhancement enterprise. The idea that a Conservative stance on biomedical enhancements would reject the enhancement enterprise is worth considering because it is more interesting than the very weak claim that enhancement is sometimes wrong, and more cogent than the very strong claim that it is never justifiable.

My aim, then, is to concentrate on concerns about enhancement that could be advanced from the distinctive perspective of the mainstream Conservative tradition, and try to see whether they amount to a compelling case against the enhancement enterprise. I will limit the inquiry to secular versions of the ideas of that tradition, for two reasons. First, as I noted in the preceding chapter, the most prominent contemporary Conservative bioethicists claim that their criticisms of enhancement need not appeal to religious doctrine. Second, my concern is to articulate the resources that the most coherent, developed Conservative thinking can bring to bear in a public debate that is accessible to religious and non-religious people alike, and that hence does not depend upon any particular religious doctrine. For the rest of this chapter, when I refer to Conservatives, I will mean those in the secular mainstream of the Burkean tradition.

My chief conclusions will be these. (1) Although Conservatism does not provide conclusive reasons either for refraining from biomedical enhancements altogether or even for not engaging in the enhancement enterprise, it does supply weighty reasons *for* developing and employing biomedical enhancements. This first, rather surprising result derives from a central thesis of Conservatism: the thesis that human nature severely constrains the possibilities for progress. If that thesis is true, and if biomedical interventions can relax these constraints, then new paths to human progress will be opened. The prospect that the very constraints that Conservatives emphasize can be relaxed undercuts the Conservative's most fundamental argument for its own superiority over doctrines of ambitious improvement. In addition, the Conservative emphasis on sustaining the goods we now enjoy provides another argument for enhancement, in circumstances in which we may need to improve our existing capacities or develop new ones to prevent the loss of what we now have and rightly value. (2) Nevertheless, Conservative thought contains three deep insights that can contribute to a reasonable pursuit of the enhancement project: the importance of continuity in the good life, the related notion that proper appreciation of existing goods is a central component of good character, and the need for humility about the reach of human knowledge, a virtue that can help reduce the risk that enhancement efforts will unwittingly disrupt benign dependences among human capacities or between human capacities and social practices and institutions. (3) The only secular version of Conservatism capable of grounding a policy of refraining from the enhancement enterprise, as opposed to pursuing it cautiously, is implausible, because it rests upon a misunderstanding of evolution—an untenable residuum of pre-Darwinian teleological biology.

As I observed in Chapter Two, enhancements are not new. Literacy, numeracy, computers (especially with the advent of the internet), as well as science, are all potent cognitive enhancements. The agrarian revolution, including the development and diffusion of agriculture and the domestication of animals, resulted in the enhancement of many human capacities—physical, social, and cognitive. I also emphasized that it is a mistake to think that these historical enhancements are different from biomedical enhancements, such as cognitive enhancement drugs or genetic engineering or tissue implants, because they do not affect human biology. Literacy and numeracy change the brain, and the agrarian revolution, the emergence of cities, and transportation technologies have changed the human genome. A better way of distinguishing biomedical from historical enhancements would be to say that the former involve interventions intended to work directly on the brain or body, based on the scientific knowledge of human biology. But from the standpoint of Conservative responses to the enhancement project—and in terms of what reflection on it can tell us about the limitations of Conservatism—what turns out to be crucial about biomedical enhancements is not their directness. It is that some of them would affect human biology in ways that call into question key Conservative assumptions about human nature.

Many different views are identified as Conservative in one domain of discourse or another. Here I'm concerned chiefly with what might be called mainstream modern Conservative thought, which originates (or at least finds its first relatively clear and most influential formulation) in the writings of Edmund Burke. Instead of attempting to state necessary and sufficient conditions for Conservatism, I'll simply consider various tenets that are uncontroversially at the core of the Conservative perspective and see what they imply about the enhancement enterprise—and how the prospect of enhancement affects *their* plausibility.

Three central conservative tenets

Three distinct tenets are prominent in the Burkean mainstream of Conservative thought. The first two are claims about human nature;

the third has to do with what Conservatives take to be a misunderstanding of human nature and society that motivates efforts at radical reform or improvement. The first is that human nature is a fixed essence created by God or Providence, as an enduring element in an overall Divine plan for the world. Call this the Created Essence View. According to this first tenet, it would be wrong to try to change human nature because to do so would be to rebel against the Divinity; hence any biomedical enhancements that would change human nature are excluded. As already noted, I won't discuss this view, because I am pursuing my subject within the constraints of secular moral reasoning and because the Conservative views I intend to scrutinize are available within both the religious and the secular currents of Conservative thought. Before proceeding farther, however, I wish to note that even if one grants the premise that human nature is a divine creation and one that the Divinity intends to have an eternal shelf life, nothing follows as to whether the enhancement project should be pursued, for the simple reason that without a lot more heavy theological lifting, one can't know when enhancement goes beyond or against human nature, and when it is simply a development of the potentials encompassed by human nature. For all we know, God's plan may include a role for us as self-improvers, and proper self-improvement, in His eyes, may include biomedical means.

The second and third Conservative tenets are both more interesting and more accessible to secular thinking. The second is that human nature includes severe and *permanent* constraints on the possibilities for human improvement through social reform. Call this the Permanent Constraint View. The third is that efforts to change human nature so as to relax these constraints are very likely to damage human life, and that such efforts are motivated by a distorted picture of humans or human society, or both. Call this the Back-Fire View. The Permanent Constraint View and the Back-Fire View are closely connected in Conservative thought: the idea is that among the permanent limitations of human nature are cognitive deficiencies that virtually guarantee the failure of human efforts to remove our natural limitations, in part because these cognitive limitations encourage a simplistic view of what improvement would require. The claim that the Permanent Constraint View and the Back-Fire View are central tenets of mainstream Conservative thought is so uncontroversial that I will not undertake the task of documenting their expression in the writings of Conservative thinkers in that tradition.[1]

According to the Permanent Constraint View, the chief constraints that human nature places on the possibilities for social reform are of two kinds: affective (motivational and emotional) and cognitive. Selfishness is prominent among the supposed motivational constraints. Thus a standard Conservative diagnosis of the root cause of the failures of State Socialism is that its proponents wrongly believed that new institutions and social practices could eliminate the need to appeal to self-interest in achieving social coordination. Emotional constraints said to be part of human nature include the dark passions of violence, overweening pride, and refusal to acknowledge rightful authority.[2] Conservatives may disagree as to the affective components of human nature, but they are unanimous in believing that humans by nature suffer from very serious *cognitive* limitations. Indeed, the emphasis on this latter type of limitation may be distinctive of mainstream Conservatism.

The most significant cognitive limitation is supposedly the human capacity for *conscious* knowledge of how to achieve mutually beneficial, stable social cooperation, which is thought to be extremely meager and to remain so. Because of this feature of human nature, attempts to construct society on a conscious plan are doomed to failure; hence, the Conservative's adamant rejection of "radical social reform." Fortunately, however, humans are capable of quite sophisticated implicit or unconscious practical knowledge. Such knowledge is built up over the centuries and is embodied in traditions, broadly understood to include institutions and social practices.

This idea of implicit or unconscious, socially embodied knowledge need not be presented in theological garb. Instead, it can be conceived naturalistically as "distributed intelligence" that emerges, without anyone willing it, through social interactions. Adam Smith's conception of the invisible hand of the market—or, more accurately, the invisible mind of the market—is a clear example. Markets embody and utilize information that no individual or group of individuals possesses.

The third Conservative tenet, the Back-Fire View, is most vividly expressed in the rejection of a particular analogy. Burke condemns radical social reformers for proceeding as if society were a simple mechanism, like a clock, capable of being produced, disassembled, and reconstituted by conscious human design.[3] Similarly, contemporary Conservative bioethicists warn that the human organism has a "precisely balanced" nature which is the result of eons of "exacting" evolution and that any attempt by mere humans to improve it is likely to end in disaster.[4] The idea is that given the limitations on conscious knowledge that human nature entails, if human beings attempt to manipulate human nature, they will wreck it; hence the title of Anthony Burgess's acclaimed dystopian novel, *A Clockwork Orange*. The point of the title is that a human being is no more a machine—a simple mechanism—than an orange is, and that attempts to improve it which do not take to heart this fundamental fact are bound to fail—and fail ruinously.

To contemporary ears, the proper response to pronouncements about human nature is caution, if not skepticism. Traditional Conservatism's naiveté about human nature is understandable; after all, this tradition developed prior to Darwin's revolution in biology. Contemporary Conservative thinkers, including Russell Kirk and Roger Scruton, tend to be as unreflective in their pronouncements about human nature (and the nature of society) as Conservative bioethicists are. They, too, proceed as if such claims were uncontroversial, steadfastly ignoring the fact that the track record on them is riddled with errors, and failing to grasp the fundamental fact that any such claims must be supported by scientific reasoning from empirical evidence.

In the preceding chapter I examined the uses and abuses of the idea of human nature in the enhancement debate, including the claim that changing our nature is wrong *per se*.[5] I concluded that whatever is valuable in appeals to human nature can be better expressed without invoking the term. Accordingly, in this chapter I will simply bracket the issues of what human nature is and how claims about it are to be justified.

It is true that Conservatives think that the cognitive and affective limitations they see in human beings are part of their nature, but what matters for the Conservative position is that these limitations are thought to be unalterable. If they were merely contingent, rather than essential features of human beings, they would still pose severe limitations on human progress, so long as they persisted. The crucial point is that Conservatives assume that these cognitive limitations *will* persist. A Conservative who abandons the idea of a fixed human nature can still adhere to the view that humans have unalterable cognitive and affective limitations that dramatically constrain the prospects of human progress through deliberate efforts at improvement.

Cognitive and affective limitations as a permanent constraint on progress

The Permanent Constraint View breaks into two claims: one about the affective limitations of human beings, the other about their cognitive limitations. What the two claims have in common is the assumption that the limitations in question are unalterable. If we avoid explanations of their existence that appeal to Providence or to some sort of secular historicist teleology that posits an ultimate goal of history, we must understand them as the product of evolutionary processes. The latter may include not only biological evolution, but also cultural evolution and co-evolution (the synergism of biological and cultural evolution, as in the emergence of lactose tolerance in dairying societies). Yet to the extent that biological evolution plays a significant role, the only reasonable prediction is unending alteration, not permanence.

It might turn out, however, that for practical purposes we may regard the cognitive and affective limitations that so impress Conservatives as fixed, when we consider undertaking radical social reforms. After all, alteration of something this fundamental, through the operation of evolutionary processes, is likely to be very slow relative to the time-horizon of human planning.[6] Even if that is true, however, it is irrelevant, because our topic is deliberate biomedical interventions, not evolution as it occurs independently of them. The prospect of biomedical enhancements that could accomplish important changes much more quickly than those brought about thus far by evolution clearly undercuts the Conservative claim that human progress is limited by unalterable constraints. If the central tenets of Conservatism only make sense on the assumption that significant relaxation of our cognitive or affective limitations could only come about very slowly, through evolution unaided by deliberate human interventions for the sake of enhancement, then Conservatism rests precariously on a dubious empirical prediction.

As the biochemical basis of motivation and emotion become better understood, our power to alter what we previously thought was our fixed nature will increase. Given that we have no good reason to assert that this power will forever fall short of significantly relaxing the emotional and motivational constraints that now exist, the Conservative begs the very question at issue by assuming that these constraints are unalterable.

Consider the Conservative assumption about unalterable cognitive limitations. This assumption also has two parts: the first is the claim that existing conscious knowledge of the workings of society and of the functioning of human beings is inadequate for purposes of making fundamental changes in either; the second is that this cognitive inadequacy will persist indefinitely.

Suppose that for now we grant the first part. The second part is sufficiently problematic to undermine the Conservative's view that we are forever incapable of deliberate radical reform or fundamental improvement. For it is simply an assertion, without argument or evidence, that human beings, because of their cognitive limitations, are incapable of incorporating knowledge that is originally a form of "distributed intelligence" into a body of conscious knowledge upon which to act. There is already one glaring counterexample to this claim: the existence of science. The social practices and traditions of the scientific community (to use language that resonates with Conservatives) include an ongoing process of identifying and assembling distributed knowledge and making it accessible as conscious, concentrated knowledge capable of guiding action. This process may never be completed: more scientific knowledge will always be available than any one scientist or groups of scientists could master. But as information technologies advance, the domain of conscious, concentrated knowledge expands. Indeed, one dramatic accomplishment of modern information technologies is that they make widely distributed knowledge available to agents in forms that can be incorporated into conscious deliberations about what to do.[7]

The Conservative's assertion that there are severe and permanent human cognitive limitations puts her in an uncomfortable position. She must show why human beings have *sufficient* cognitive power to know that their cognitive powers are severely limited *and* to know that the traditional social arrangements embody superior knowledge, but *insufficient* cognitive power to overcome those limitations. More specifically, the Conservative claim that the tacit knowledge embodied in traditional social arrangements is—and will remain—superior to anything that human beings could ever come to know consciously is a sweeping empirical claim. If we avoid appeals to Providence, it is a claim that must be supported by work in the social sciences—an anecdotal and highly selective reading of history will not suffice. But to assert that it can be so supported is to admit that conscious knowledge of how society works is quite impressive. And that admission should erode the

Conservative's confidence that we will never know enough to undertake significant social reform without disastrous consequences.

This tension in the Conservative's view about cognitive limitations becomes much more troubling when we add to the possibility of advances in social science the prospect of cognitive enhancements by biomedical means. How could anyone at this point in time, when biomedical enhancements are just becoming practicable, be in a position to predict that human beings whose cognitive powers are enhanced by a combination of biomedical and nonbiomedical technologies (such as improved computers) will not significantly exceed our current conscious knowledge of how society works?

Of course, the Conservative could reply that he is not wedded to any such extravagantly pessimistic prediction, that instead his point is simply that *for now* the cognitive limitations of human beings preclude deliberate large-scale improvements. That claim is certainly more plausible, but it dramatically deflates the Conservative view: it renders Conservatism incapable of providing a compelling reason against pursuing the enhancement enterprise as opposed to pursuing it cautiously. Pursuing the enhancement enterprise does *not* mean attempting radical social reform or radical biological modification. It means recognizing biomedical enhancement as a legitimate end for individuals, as an appropriate policy goal, and as a sufficiently controversial and risky undertaking to warrant ongoing public deliberation and institutional controls. Endorsing the enhancement enterprise does not commit one to hubristic assumptions about the scope of feasible improvement or about how rapidly improvements can be made.

The argument thus far can now be summarized. There is good reason to believe that the cognitive, emotional, and motivational constraints on progress that Conservatives emphasize can be significantly relaxed by biotechnology or by a combination of biotechnology and the growth of scientific knowledge, including knowledge of how society works. The strongest reason for believing that the cognitive limitations of human beings are not fixed is that we have already enhanced our cognitive capacities dramatically—through literacy, numeracy, science, and electronic, digitalized information technologies. A striking feature of these cognitive enhancements is that they have extended the domain of concentrated, conscious knowledge. In each case, cognitive enhancement technology allows many minds to contribute to bodies of knowledge far more extensive and complex than any individual mind could have produced, but then also makes that knowledge accessible to many individual minds.

There are two weighty reasons for believing that our emotional and motivational capacities are not fixed either. The first is that they are at least in significant part the product of biological evolution, and biological evolution is not capable of producing anything that is unalterable. The second is that we have already begun to understand the biochemical basis of emotion and motivation sufficiently well to allow its manipulation, as evidenced by some rather dramatic successes in altering the affective behavior of laboratory animals and, to a lesser extent, in the widespread use of mood-altering drugs in humans. Thus we have no good reason to assume that our current cognitive and affective limitations are fixed; and we certainly should not be *so* confident that they are as to appeal to their supposed fixity as a reason for refraining from the enhancement project. If this is so, then it is viciously circular to argue that we should not undertake the enhancement project because all attempts to achieve significant progress are doomed by the unalterable cognitive and affective constraints to which human beings are currently subject.

The unsupported assumption that human beings have unalterable cognitive and affective features that constitute severe limitations on human progress is the Achilles heel of Conservatism—and not just with regard to Conservative opposition to biomedical enhancement. Once the assumption of unalterability is called into doubt, the most distinctively Conservative argument against efforts to achieve fundamental improvements in human affairs, whether through deliberate social reform or biomedical technologies or some combination of the two, simply collapses. Conservatives are quite right to emphasize that any project of fundamental reform or significant improvement must take feasibility into account, but that cannot rule out efforts, such as the enhancement enterprise, to remove some of the constraints that presently determine what is feasible.

Genetically engineered versus clockwork oranges

We have seen that the second core Conservative tenet, the Permanent Constraint View, is incapable of supporting either the general thesis that efforts at fundamental improvements in the human condition are forever doomed to failure, or the particular thesis that we should abstain from the enhancement enterprise. I now want to argue that the third Conservative tenet, the Back-Fire View, is equally problematic and is also incapable of grounding a rejection of the enhancement enterprise. The Back-Fire View is the claim that a perilously inapt analogy drives efforts for radical reform or fundamental human improvement: the clock or simple machine analogy.

No one who possesses even a minimal understanding of modern biological science in general or of genomics in particular thinks that oranges, much less human beings, are much like machines, even complicated machines, let alone that they are like clocks. Other analogies (all with their limitations, of course) are much more appealing, including the computer analogy or, more broadly, the idea of a complex, imperfectly self-regulating information-processing system (or collection of such systems, ranging from the computational brain to the epigenome) that both responds to and acts on its environment. So, if the Conservative's perennial appeal to the machine or clock analogies is to do the argumentative work it is intended to do, the claim must *not* be that, as an enterprise that is reasonably informed by modern science, the enhancement project is driven by such absurdly oversimplified analogies. Instead, the Conservative's claim must be that no matter how much more sophisticated our knowledge becomes, any attempt to use it to effect significant alterations of ourselves or our social institutions will betray an unacceptably risky underestimation of how complex the objects of our interventions are. Call this the Conservative's *iron law of hubris*.[8]

What are we to make of it? It is an empirical prediction of staggering proportions and one for which neither Conservatives nor anybody else has offered scientifically respectable evidence. Clearly, the iron law of hubris is not the sort of thing one can support by intuition or anecdote or vague, nonquantitative, impressionistic reflections on history. If we set aside the theological claims that some Conservatives make about human nature, we are left with a very strong empirical prediction, bereft of anything like adequate evidence.[9] The weaker and more qualified the prediction of dangerous hubris becomes, the more plausible it is; but only a very strong and unqualified prediction could ground the conclusion that we ought not to pursue the enhancement project, and adequate evidence for that sort of prediction is conspicuously absent.

Unwitting disruption of benign dependencies

A related claim *is* highly plausible, however, namely, that there is a serious risk that our desire for improvement will outstrip our knowledge of how to bring it about. One well-known source of this discrepancy between the desire for improvement and the ability to bring it about is the error of not taking feasibility seriously enough in deciding what to aim for. But there is another, equally important failing: the risk of unintended bad consequences and, more specifically, the risk of *unwittingly disrupting benign dependencies*. The simple and important idea here is that, because of the *connectedness* of what we wish to alter with what we wish to preserve, we may do great harm in trying to enhance.

One example among many will illustrate this risk. It is widely reported that substantial numbers of college students, especially at elite US institutions, are taking prescription drugs to enhance normal cognitive performance.[10] The safety of such "off-label" use of drugs has not been established. It may turn out that we will come to identify a serious adverse reaction, but only after a period of prolonged use of a particular drug by many individuals, and only after irreparable damage has been done. One possibility is that the price of the cognitive enhancements these drugs achieve is the disruption of some other cognitive function or of some affective functions.

The worry about unwitting disruption of benign dependencies can and should be voiced without buying into the Conservative's iron law of hubris. The worry can be adequately captured by an unblinking attention to past cases of technological overreach, along with an understanding of the sorts of situations in which there are strong incentives for overestimating the benefits of innovations and underestimating the harms. Some of the most notorious historical cases are interventions to solve one problem that have created equally serious ones, due to ignorance of connections within ecological systems. Among the most obvious incentives that can encourage technological overreach are the interests of putative experts in convincing others and sometimes themselves that their expertise is greater than it in fact is.[11]

Given the potential benefits of enhancement, some of which I explored in Chapter Two,[12] the reasonable approach is to try to develop norms and institutions to reduce this risk of unintended bad consequences, not to refrain from the enhancement project altogether.[13] A complete ban on enhancements, no matter how great the benefits they might bring, might make sense if connectedness was *so extreme* that any intervention carried an unacceptable risk of unintended bad consequences. In Chapter Four I noted that the critics of enhancement provide no evidence to support the extreme connectedness assumption. In the next two sections of this chapter, I argue that evolutionary biology gives us good reason to reject it.

The implausibility of an absolute prohibition on biomedical enhancement, as a response to the risk of unintended bad consequences, becomes all the more obvious once we recognize just how manifold the enhancement project is. Some attempted enhancements (such as genetic modifications of human embryos) may be much riskier than others (such as highly controlled, closely monitored trials of cognitive enhancement drugs on informed, consenting adults). The central point, however, is that there are better ways of grounding the admonition to take seriously the risk of unwitting disruption of benign interdependencies than by swallowing extravagant views about the permanent limitations of human nature, the iron law of hubris, or the implausible assertion that absurdly oversimplified machine analogies are driving the pursuit of enhancement.[14]

So, absent support for the extreme connectedness assumption, the Conservative idea that humans suffer severe cognitive and affective limitations does not provide a good reason to refrain from all enhancements, and in fact counts heavily in favor of pursuing those enhancements that would remove or ameliorate these limitations. Nor does it warrant the conclusion that we should not pursue the enhancement enterprise, so long as we do so in a way that takes proper account of our *current* limitations and the risks they may pose to our efforts to remove them. In Chapter Six, I offer a set of cautionary heuristics, informed by evolutionary biology, that are designed to reduce the risks that the current limitations of biological knowledge will result in bad unintended consequences if we attempt enhancements involving inheritable genetic modifications of humans.

The analogy of the Master Engineer of evolution

I now want to argue that those same Conservative bioethicists who bemoan the simple machine analogy themselves employ an analogy that betrays gross misunderstandings of how evolution works, when they suggest that efforts at biomedical enhancement are doomed to failure. The Conservative bioethicists' analogy is that of evolution as a *Master Engineer.* Consider again the assertion, cited earlier, that "The human body and mind, highly complex and delicately balanced as the result of eons of gradual and exacting evolution, are almost certainly at risk from any ill-considered attempt at 'improvement.'. . ."

Notice that the Conservatives who make this assertion, unlike more traditional Conservatives like Burke, avoid any suggestion that the human organism is the product of Divine design. Instead, they appeal to the idea that it is a product of evolution. But their conception of evolution is profoundly mistaken. They think of the evolved organism as "delicately balanced," a fragile *fait accompli*, a finished product created by a Master Engineer—that is, a *stable, completed masterpiece* that can only be ruined by any human attempt to improve it.[15]

According to modern evolutionary biology, no type of organism is stable and the idea of completeness is entirely inapplicable. In fact, there is mounting evidence that Darwinian competition occurs not only between organisms, but also *within* them, including at the level of genes.[16] More importantly, to analogize the evolutionary process with the work of a Master Engineer is exceedingly misleading. First, a Master Engineer makes something according to a plan: he imagines a product and then goes about producing it. By contrast, in evolution there is no plan. That is why even Richard Dawkins's famous analogy of the "blind watchmaker" is far too charitable. (A blind watchmaker knows what he is trying to produce, namely, a watch, something intended to satisfy human desires or needs.) Second, evolution does not produce harmonious, flawless objects: it cobbles together unstable products, the majority of which are destroyed rather quickly and all of which eventually break down.

The fact that natural selection *has* operated on a trait does not ensure that the trait *is* optimal.[17] "Adaptation," in the most uncontroversial sense, refers to *how* a trait came to fixation in a population, *not* to its *current* conduciveness to reproductive fitness. Optimality, if it ever exists (as opposed to being approximated) is fleeting, because the environment of adaptation is constantly shifting. This is vividly conveyed by the famous Red Queen Hypothesis, according to which organisms have to keep running faster just to stay where they are (i.e., they must adapt merely to maintain their present fitness levels) as the selective environment crumbles beneath their feet.

It is worth recalling that it was Darwin's growing appreciation of how *unlike* the products of a Master Engineer all living things are that prompted him to develop his theory. Recall his letter to Joseph Hooker, from which I quoted in Chapter One: "What a book a Devil's Chaplain might write on the clumsy, wasteful, blundering low and horridly cruel works of nature."[18] Examples of poor biological design abound: the urinary tract in male mammals, which passes through (rather than around) the prostate gland, and which consequently is prone to blockage if the gland swells, leading to infection and loss of urinary function; the primate sinus, which has a feeble drainage system, also leading to infection, discomfort and in some cases chronic pain; the inability of humans to biosynthesize vitamin C due to a mutation which most other mammals do not have and which appears to confer no benefit whatsoever, and which has led over the course of mankind's existence to widespread, debilitating disease and countless deaths; the blind spot in the vertebrate eye (resulting from quirks of embryological development), which forces vertebrates to develop elaborate and costly perception-correcting mechanism; the human pharynx, whose dual function of both ingestion of food and respiration significantly increases the risk of death by choking; the birth canal in humans passing through the pelvis, which dramatically increases the dangers of childbirth, thanks to selection's hasty rearrangement of hominid posture with the advent of bipedalism (along with the increase in cranial size); and the propensity for lower back pain and disability that resulted when a knuckle-walking ape became a bipedal hominid. The list goes on and on, for both the human and every other species.

Given the way evolution works, it is utterly predictable that design flaws, departures from what a Master Engineer would produce, will be ubiquitous. In brief, evolution *inevitably* produces suboptimal designs. The clumsy, wasteful, blundering forms that so impressed Darwin are not perturbations in the process, they are essential to it; that is precisely his point.

There is another fundamental fact about evolution that even further undercuts the usefulness of appealing to it in the way that Conservatives do in arguments against the enhancement project: what natural selection approximates (and then, only fleetingly, as we have seen) is reproductive fitness, *not what human beings rightly value*. So even if (contrary to the facts of evolutionary biology) the human organism were a "finely balanced," stable, finished product, there is no reason to believe that it is optimal from the standpoint of what *we* care about.

The best that can be said for the Conservative's Master Engineer analogy is that it is a misleading way of expressing a more commonsensical concern that can be adequately expressed without reliance on distorted views about evolution. Evolution does produce highly complex organisms. Given this complexity—and note that "complexity" does not mean "harmony," "goodness," or "delicate balance" either within the human individual or between humans and the environment—we ought to take very seriously the risk of unwittingly disrupting benign dependencies. That is what I do in the next chapter. Here I want to focus on the uses of metaphors in Conservative thinking and their implications for enhancement.

Switching Conservative analogies: the House of Cards

Perhaps the Conservative has a rejoinder, a different analogy to be enlisted in the cause of anti-enhancement arguments, based on a *rejection* of the Master Engineer analogy.[19] Given our current cognitive limitations, attempts to use biotechnologies to overcome our current cognitive limitations are very likely to produce disastrous results *because* evolution is *not* like a Master Engineer. If it were like a Master Engineer, our limited intellects would be more capable of understanding its products precisely because its products would make more sense. Because evolution's products are riddled with design flaws, unplanned, and cobbled together using severely constrained biological resources, our efforts to modify them are all the more likely to go awry. The idea here is that because masterful design exhibits simplicity and efficiency, less intelligence is required to understand the works of a Master Engineer than the unnecessarily complex, inefficient, Rube Goldberg products of evolution. The products of evolution are not "finely balanced" as a result of masterful design, but because they are so poorly designed they are exceedingly fragile. What we think will be a limited change that will be beneficial may cause the House of Cards to collapse.

Abandoning the Master Engineer analogy in favor of the House of Cards analogy doesn't help matters from a Conservative point of view. *If the human organism is so poorly designed as to be exceedingly fragile, then we may need to improve it if we are to survive.* If we are as fragile as the

House of Cards analogy suggests, we are already in a very risky situation. If we are "finely balanced" in the way a House of Cards is, then even relatively small changes in the environment may cause collapse. Even worse, because human beings have developed powerful technologies, other actions we undertake that have nothing to do with enhancement may cause the House of Cards to collapse. Once we recognize that our interventions for the sake of enhancement are not the only things that can cause the House of Cards to collapse, we have to take seriously the possibility that the most rational response to the perils of fragility is to develop the ability to make ourselves less fragile. Instead of waiting for some environmental change or unwitting effect of human action to cause the House of Cards to collapse, shouldn't we start figuring out ways to shore it up? The House of Cards analogy, then, seems to point us toward the opposite of a Conservative conclusion: if the analogy is accurate, we can't afford to leave things as they are.

It would be a mistake, however, to rely on this analogy in trying to decide how to respond to the possibilities of enhancement. The House of Cards analogy is not well supported by evolutionary biology. The human organism, like all other organisms, includes some systems and subsystems that are quite ancient, having been conserved with relatively little change since they first appeared in our distant ancestors. These conserved features exist alongside more recent features. In some cases the newer features result in *redundancy*; in other cases both the new and the old perform important functions but operate in relatively independent fashion. Given the combination of conserved and newly emerging systems and subsystems that characterizes evolution, it is not surprising that redundancy is pervasive. To the extent that redundancy limits fragility, the House of Cards analogy is inaccurate and misleading.

In addition to redundancy, the pervasiveness of *modularity* in biology discredits the Seamless Web analogy. Modifying one module need not alter other systems and subsystems. Modularity in embryonic development creates "developmental firewalls" in this sense: if something goes wrong in one module, the damage may be contained within that module.[20]

Along with redundancy and modularization, *canalization* is a third feature of organisms that undermines the credibility of the House of Cards and Seamless Web as guiding analogies for thinking intelligently about the risks of biomedical enhancement. Canalization is the tendency of a developmental system to produce a particular phenotype notwithstanding variations in genotype or environment. The stronger the canalization, the less liable to variation—that is, the less "fragile"—the phenotype is in the face of genetic or environmental changes, including those we might produce by our enhancement efforts.[21] Genetic redundancy is one of the principal mechanisms of canalization: if one copy of a gene mutates, there may be no adverse consequence if other copies remain.[22]

Modularity limits connectedness: by definition a module is a subsystem that has greater connectedness among its constituents than between it and other subsystems. Redundancy and canalization take some of the sting out of connectedness. If altering a characteristic severs its connection with something else of value, this need not be a problem if there is a back-up connection. Canalization means that there is more than one way to reach a developmental endpoint, so unwittingly disrupting one route need not prevent the organism from safely arriving at the destination.

Indeed, one of the fundamental differences in structural design between living things and machines is the robustness of organisms compared to the brittleness of machines when it comes to the modification of their component systems.[23] The fact that there is considerable evidence against extreme connectedness should not be surprising from an evolutionary standpoint. An organism characterized by extreme connectedness would be extraordinarily fragile in the face of environmental changes and mutations. Seamless webs and houses of cards would not be likely to survive the rigors of natural selection.

Abandoning the Master Engineer analogy (because it grossly misunderstands evolution) has two important implications for the enhancement debate. First, as I argued in Chapter Four, it undercuts Conservative "arguments" against enhancement based on the assumption that the natural is good. Second, if we abandon the Master Engineer analogy and take evolutionary biology seriously, *we must acknowledge that evolved organisms are not stable, finished products whose continued existence is threatened only by human interventions.* We must consider the possibility that human interventions may be required for the continued existence of species, whether they be human or nonhuman. Persistence is not the default position for organisms. So, it is wrong to assume that all will be well if we can only resist the temptation to intervene in our biology.

There is a grain of truth in the House of Cards analogy, however. We should not underestimate the difficulty of figuring out the causal interdependencies in an organism that is patched together in the way we are. Acknowledging this difficulty and the risk it entails is a great distance, however, from concluding that we should try to abstain from biomedical enhancements altogether or even that we should not embark on the enhancement enterprise.

The argument from biological and social harmony

A sober appreciation of what evolution is like also saps the force of another Conservative argument that is closely related to the argument that we should not try to improve on the work of the Master Engineer. Call this the Argument from Biological and Social Harmony. The idea is that human biology and social institutions are in complex, balanced harmony, so that efforts to change the former may dangerously disrupt the latter. Thus, for example, Conservative bioethicists such as Leon Kass proclaim that biomedical enhancements of human reproductive capacities, such as nuclear transfer (Dolly-style) cloning, could undermine the institutions of marriage and the family and the goods that depend upon them.[24]

This argument contains a grain of truth, but not one large enough to ground the conclusion that we should refrain from the enhancement project. It helpfully elaborates the worry about unwittingly disrupting benign dependencies by pointing out that the social institutions we have are connected with our biology in ways we do not fully understand. But where the argument goes wrong is in assuming that there is a fragile, stable, harmony between social institutions and human biology. Existing human biology undoubtedly constrains the feasible set of social arrangements, but that does not mean that our biology and our institutions are in harmony, nor that any attempt to change some aspects of our biology is likely to cause unacceptable disruptions of our institutions. There is no good reason to think that remedying our inability to biosynthesize vitamin C or enhancing our immune systems or supplementing mechanical joint replacement technology with regenerative stem cell technology or extending the human life span by 20 years or increasing average IQ by 10 points would cause unacceptable social disruption. (It is worth recalling that human life expectancy has risen far more than that since 1900 and that there has been a significant rise in average IQ over the last 50 years—the so-called Flynn Effect—but this has not resulted in the social fabric unraveling.)

Predictions of social disruptions are just that: predictions. If we are to appeal to such predictions as reasons for forgoing biomedical enhancements that are of great potential benefit, we need credible evidence for the predictions. Those who make them never seem to present evidence or even to acknowledge the need for evidence. In the next chapter, I consider a possible rejoinder to this demand for evidence: the view that if the magnitude of the harm that a biomedical enhancement might cause is great, then we are justified in prohibiting the enhancement, even if we lack substantial evidence that the harm is not merely possible, but likely to occur. There I examine the relevance of the Precautionary Principle for the ethics of biomedical enhancement. The point I wish to make here is simply that there is no area of human life in which the mere possibility of a cost is a good reason for refraining from an action that is reasonably expected to bring considerable benefit. In previous chapters I have argued that there is no reason to think that biomedical enhancement is an exception to this general rule.

Conserving existing goods through enhancement

Accepting the rosy picture of a stable harmonious relationship between human biology and social institutions may in fact be dangerous. Given the plausible assumption that cultural evolution generally produces change much more rapidly than biological evolution, it would not be surprising if there were cases where our biological evolution has not kept up with the new problems our cultural evolution has produced. Most evolutionary biologists think that the distinctive features of human biology emerged in response to the demands of the Environment of Ancestral Adaptedness (EAA), which they take to have existed in the Pleistocene Era, between 40 and 200 thousand years ago. Since that time, there have been changes, for example through natural selection for disease resistance and for reduced pigmentation in more northerly climates, but our basic equipment is pretty much the same.

Given how much our present environment differs from the EAA, we may need to undertake particular enhancements to solve the culturally produced problems that our biological evolution cannot solve or cannot solve quickly enough if disaster is to be averted. In order to cope with some of the environmental problems our cultural evolution has produced, it may be necessary, among other strategies, to employ biomedical enhancements—perhaps to improve the body's capacity for thermal regulation under conditions of global warming, or to alter skin cells so that they have greater resistance to skin cancer if the ozone layer further depletes, or to sustain adequate fertility if environmental toxins drastically lower sperm counts. More ambitiously, it may be necessary to enhance human beings morally—for example, by improving their capacities for empathy and moral imagination—in a world in which new technologies give even a handful of individuals the capacity to inflict great harm.[25]

Consider another possibility: if an emerging infectious disease becomes a global pandemic, thanks to modern transportation technologies and the rather recent density of human settlements, the result could be a significant loss of human genetic diversity. Natural selection, in this case in the form of a lethal disease, acts as a filter for genes—it reduces genetic diversity. When natural selection pressures are extremely robust, as in an extremely virulent pandemic with an extraordinarily high case mortality rate, much genetic diversity will be lost. Under these circumstances, it might be necessary to enhance normal human reproductive capacities to reliably restore genetic diversity and to do so within a reasonable time frame. The millions of human tissue samples already in storage could provide the DNA to be reintroduced into the human gene pool. This, too, would be an enhancement (of normal human reproductive capacities), but one which was used, not to improve human well-being above the status quo, but to help secure it.

These last examples illustrate a more fundamental problem with any attempt to appeal to Conservative tenets as a reason for abstaining from the enhancement project as opposed to pursuing it cautiously. As I noted earlier Tancredi, in Lampedusa's brilliant novel, *The Leopard*—perhaps the best fictional exploration of the meaning of Conservatism we possess—says that if everything is to remain the same, everything will have to change. Tancredi's point is well taken. To avoid losing some of the good things we now enjoy, we will have to enhance ourselves in particular ways. To the extent that we take seriously the idea that Conservatism emphasizes conserving what is valuable, we ought to avoid the error of thinking that Conservation precludes enhancement and acknowledge that it may in fact require it. We may need further cognitive enhancements, in the form of

better computer hardware and software or biomedical cognitive enhancements, or some combination of the two, to avert the calamities of global
warming, for example. This point by itself, quite apart from the other
considerations I have offered, shows that Conservatism is incapable of
taking the enhancement enterprise off the table.

A proper appreciation of existing good

Some liberals might be surprised to know that prominent Conservatives
assert that Conservatism is the philosophy of *enjoyment*. That assertion is
perfectly accurate: Conservatism emphasizes the importance of enjoying
and valuing the good things that now exist, where this entails taking pains
to preserve them, including the cultivation of a presumption against
endangering them through the pursuit of novelty or even of things
thought to have greater value. To use the terminology of Chapter Two,
Conservatives think that the virtue of appreciation is an important constituent of good character. They also believe that societies in which this
virtue is widespread will be better in a number of ways—more stable,
more harmonious, more enriched by continuity between generations, etc.

This Conservative insight is extremely valuable. The question, however, is this: What are its practical implications for biomedical enhancement? I will not repeat my attempt to answer this question in Chapter
Two. Instead, I will only summarize my conclusion: due regard for the
virtue of appreciation should be factored in to our personal and collective deliberations about enhancement, but it cannot ground either the
conclusion that we should refrain from enhancements altogether or that
we should not undertake the enhancement enterprise, for two reasons.
First, enhancement may be needed to preserve the goods we now enjoy
(Tancredi's point); second, any reasonable presumption in favor of
preserving existing value can be overridden, if the benefits of change
are great enough, and recognizing this is compatible with the realization
that the mere fact that a change would produce more value than the
status quo is often not a sufficient reason for change.

The value of continuity

Conservatives tend to stress the importance of continuity in human life.
Sometimes "continuity" is used simply as a cognate for "incrementalism,"

and the distrust of radical change that lies at the core of Conservatism is typically accompanied by confidence in incremental change as the path to improvement. This is a significant point, because it is wrong to saddle Conservatives with the view that change is always bad—or that it is avoidable.

Conservative thought encompasses an emphasis on continuity that cannot be reduced to its advocacy of incrementalism, however. Intergenerational continuity, according to Conservatives, is of crucial importance, because human good depends upon the integration of individuals into an intergenerational community. "Integration" here includes identification: a good human life is one in which the individual thinks of herself and lives her life as a member of a collective that includes, in Burke's words, the dead, the living, and the yet unborn.

On its least problematic interpretation, this emphasis on continuity is simply an empirical psychological claim: individuals will experience alienation or a sense of purposeless or at least will not find life as good as it could be, if they identify only with their contemporaries. As such, it is both intuitively plausible and of direct relevance to the enhancement project. Suppose that major enhancements were introduced through genetically engineering the offspring of a sizeable cohort of young adults, with the result that the children of this generation were quite different from their parents, affectively, cognitively, and even physically. Suppose also that these differences allowed them to engage in relationships with each other that were unavailable to the unenhanced,[26] Isn't it possible that these new individuals and their children and so on would regard themselves as so different from the unenhanced generations that preceded them that they would not be capable of identifying with them as fully as we are now capable of identifying with our forebears?

That scenario may be unrealistic. Enhancements are more likely to come about over a more extended period of time, rather than through a one-off intervention, as the technologies develop and gain acceptance. Furthermore, large-scale genetic engineering of human embryos may be a long way off. Perhaps a better thought experiment is to imagine that the cumulative result of many generations of various enhancements is a human population that is significantly different from it predecessors. If the accumulation of individually incremental enhancements reached a "tipping point," then perhaps it would make identification more difficult. In the most extreme case, the new, enhanced people might regard those who came before them as "primitives" or even as "not yet humans."

I do not wish to dismiss the worry about loss of identification through radical change. I would like to point out, however, that there is some reason to believe that to the extent that they are greatly enhanced, future generations would be in a good position to understand their predecessors much better than we understand ours and yet would still have a rather broad basis for identification with them. If future generations are cognitively and affectively enhanced, and benefit from much more advanced work in history and social psychology, then presumably they will be able to see that they still share some fundamental characteristics and values with their predecessors. For example, even if they live to be 400 years old, they will still be mortal, like us, and they will be better able to appreciate the implications of this shared mortality because of the enhancements they enjoy. They might also identify with us as fellow participants in the enhancement enterprise or, more generally, in the broader endeavor of improving the human condition, striving for justice, etc. Many differences are compatible with the persistence of valuable identifications.

So far I have been trying to be as charitable as possible to the worry about loss of continuity. In doing so, I have focused on possible long-term consequences of the most extreme sort of enhancements, including genetic engineering of human embryos. To keep the worry about loss of continuity in perspective, however, it is important to note that for the foreseeable future, enhancements are not likely to undermine the capacity for the more valuable intergenerational identifications. Beings that live somewhat longer than we do, that are somewhat more intelligent than we are, less prone to some of the infirmities of old age than we are, physically stronger and quicker than we are, and somewhat better able to control destructive emotions than we are would still be recognizably human in the sense relevant to the most basic sort of identification.

Without much more solid empirical knowledge than we now possess about the conditions under which valuable intergenerational identification can exist, it is hard to know how serious the risk of loss of continuity is and just how an appreciation of it should inform our receptiveness to the enhancement project. The most the Conservative can plausibly say on this matter is that if we choose to pursue the enhancement enterprise we should try to learn more about the conditions of valuable intergenerational identifications and, on the basis of that knowledge, take whatever steps are necessary to reduce the risk to levels that are commensurate with the expected benefits of various enhancements. For if generations in the distant future rightly believed that their quality of life was dramatically better than ours, then they might rightly conclude that that although the loss of a sense of shared identity with their predecessors was a genuine loss, it was an acceptable one.

Conclusion

The motivation for this chapter was a sense that critiques of enhancement by Conservative bioethicists are confused and superficial—that they are not grounded in a coherent moral–political view. My aim, accordingly, was to ascertain whether traditional, mainstream Conservative thought can provide better insights about enhancement. The results of the inquiry have been surprising. Indeed, to some they will be shocking. The prospect of biomedical enhancement undercuts a key premise in the Conservative's argument against radical improvement, the thesis that human beings suffer severe cognitive and affective limitations. If these limitations are as debilitating as Conservatives say they are, and if enhancements can alleviate them, then the quintessentially Conservative emphasis on human beings' imperfections provides a reason in favor of enhancement, rather than against it. In addition, the Conservative emphasis on the importance of sustaining the goods we now enjoy can speak in favor of enhancement, because we may need to enhance some of our capacities to avoid losing goods we now have.

The Conservative themes of epistemic humility, of a proper appreciation of the goods we now possess, and of continuity as an element of the good life are critical resources for devising a responsible approach to enhancement. But in the end, the implications that Conservatism has for biomedical enhancement may be less interesting than the implications of biomedical enhancement for Conservatism. The more robust our ability to change ourselves becomes, the less plausible the attempt to develop a moral and political vision based on the assumption that human nature is a permanent and severe limitation on the possibility of progress.

Notes

1. For an informative, though partisan, exploration of the writings of major contributors to the mainstream, Burkean tradition of Conservative thought, see Russell Kirk (2001), *The Conservative Mind: From Burke to Eliot*, 7th edn., revised (Washington, DC: Regnery Publishing).
2. Using language that is perhaps more congenial to traditional Conservatives, these may also be called moral imperfections.
3. Citing Burke, Kirk (2001: 45) writes: "Prejudice and prescription, despite their great age—or, rather, because of it – are delicate growths, slow to rise, easy to injure, hardly possible to resuscitate. The abstract metaphysician and fanatic reformer, intending to cleanse society, may find he has scrubbed it clean away: An ignorant man, who is not fool enough to meddle with his clock, is however sufficiently confident to think he can safely take to pieces, and put together at his pleasure, a moral machine of another guise, importance, and complexity, composed of far other wheels, and springs, and balances, and counter-acting and co-operating powers . . . Their delusive good intention is no sort of excuse for their presumption." Endnote 29: "Appeal from the New Whigs," *Works*, III, pp. 111–112.
4. President's Council on Bioethics (2002), *Beyond Therapy* (Washington, DC: National Bioethics Advisory Commission).
5. See also Allen Buchanan (2009), "Human Nature and Enhancement," *Bioethics*, 23: 141–150.
6. How plausible that assumption is will depend, *inter alia*, on the relative strengths of biological and cultural evolution, given the reasonable hypothesis that significant change can occur much more quickly through cultural evolution than through biological evolution.
7. Just as important, the Conservative's strong separation between tacit, distributed social knowledge and conscious, concentrated knowledge is an exaggeration, as the case of markets illustrates. Whether the invisible mind of the market operates properly depends in part upon regulations and other interventions in it that are guided by conscious, concentrated knowledge, above all, knowledge of how the market, as a system of tacit, distributed knowledge operates.
8. Albert O. Hirschman (1991) insightfully explores the role of "iron laws" in Conservative thinking in *The Rhetoric of Reaction: Perversity, Futility, Jeopardy* (Cambridge: The Belknap Press).
9. It is worth noting that, if anything, my critique of Conservative views of human nature thus far has been too charitable. I have conceded, *arguendo*, the central Conservative claim that human nature includes severe motivational and emotional constraints on the possibilities for improvement. But the Conservative's account of what human nature is like is problematic, even if it is understood simply as a description of the way we are, not as a claim about essences. The Conservative view of human characteristics tends to be

more anecdotal than scientific and to ignore relevant scientific findings that seem to contradict them. For example, to the extent that the Conservative view includes the idea that human beings are by nature violently asocial (and that only the constraining and tutoring functions of tradition civilize us), it is vulnerable to scientific findings that stress the biologically evolved sociability of primates. See, for example, Franz de Waal (2006), *Primates and Philosophers: How Morality Evolved*, S. Macedo, J. Ober (eds.) (Princeton: Princeton University Press) for an empirical critique of the view that humans are "naturally" asocial.

10. On the non-medical use of prescription stimulants among US college students, see Sean Esteban McCabe, John R. Knight, Christian J. Teter and Henry Wechsler (2005), "Non-medical use of prescription stimulants among US college students: prevalence and correlates from a national survey," *Addiction* 99: 96–106.

11. Allen Buchanan (1996), "Is There a Medical Profession in the House," in *Conflicts of Interest in Clinical Practice and Research*, David Schimm *et al.* (eds.) (Oxford: Oxford University Press), pp. 105–136; and Allen Buchanan (1996), "Toward a Theory of the Ethics of Bureaucratic Organizations," *Business Ethics Quarterly*, 6: 419–440. Geoffrey Brennan and Alan Hamlin (2004), "Analytic Conservatism," *British Journal of Political Science* 34: 675–692.

12. See also Allen Buchanan (forthcoming), "Enhancement and the Ethics of Development," *Kennedy Institute Journal of Ethics* 18: 1–34.

13. It is generally assumed that the risk of unintended bad consequences is greatest in the case of germline genetic modifications. For a proposal of a set of cautionary heuristics for reducing this risk, grounded in an accurate understanding of modern evolutionary biology, see Russell Powell and Allen Buchanan (forthcoming), "Breaking Evolution's Chains: The Promise of Enhancement By Design," Ruud ter Muelen, Julian Savulescu, and Guy Kahane (eds.) *Enhancing Human Capacities* (Oxford: Oxford University Press).

14. Ibid.

15. Much of the remainder of this section is drawn from Powell and Buchanan forthcoming, *supra* note 13.

16. For a discussion of intergenic competition within a single organism, see, for example, Richard Dawkins (1976), *The Selfish Gene* (Oxford: Oxford University Press); Egbert Giles Leigh, Jr. (1971), *Adaptation and Diversity: Natural History and the Mathematics of Evolution* (San Francisco: Freeman, Cooper & Company), Chapter 15; Elliott Sober (1984), *The Nature of Selection: Evolutionary Theory in Philosophical Focus* (Cambridge, MA: MIT Press), Chapters 7–9. For discussion of intercellular competition within a single organism, see Leo Buss (1987), *The Evolution of Individuality* (Princeton: Princeton University Press).

170   *Conservatism and Enhancement*

17. For a lengthy treatment of the issue of optimality in evolution, see Richard Dawkins (1999), *The Extended Phenotype: The Long Reach of the Gene* (Oxford: Oxford University Press), Chapter 3.
18. Quoted in R. Dawkins (2004), *A Devil's Chaplain: Reflection on Hope, Lies, Science, and Love* (Mariner Books), p. 8.
19. I thank Kai Hirutu and Tony Cole for suggesting this point.
20. See C.P. Klingenberg (2008), "Morphological Integration and Development of Modularity," *Annual Review of Ecological Evolutionary Systems* 39: 115–132.
21. See G. Gibson and G. Wagner (2000), "Canalization in evolutionary genetics: a stabilizing theory?" *Bioessays* 22(4): 372–380.
22. I am grateful to David Crawford and Russell Powell for their input on the topic of canalization in biology.
23. S. Ciliberti, O. Martin, and A. Wagner (2007), "Innovation and robustness in complex regulatory gene networks," *PNAS* 104: 13591–13596.
24. President's Council on Bioethics (2002), *Human Cloning and Human Dignity: An Ethical Inquiry* (Washington, DC: National Bioethics Advisory Commission), pp. 68–75.
25. Ingmar Persson and Julian Savulescu (2008), "The Perils of Cognitive Enhancement and the Urgent Imperative to Enhance the Moral Character of Humanity," *Journal of Applied Philosophy* 25(3): 162–177.
26. For an exploration of the implications of such a scenario for conceptions of equal rights and equal moral status, see Allen Buchanan, "Moral Status and Enhancement," Philosophy & Public Affairs, vol . 37, No. 4, 2009, pp. 346–381.

CHAPTER SIX

Unintended Bad Consequences

The problem of risk

Thus far I've argued that there is nothing morally amiss about enhancement as such, including biomedical enhancement. Neither efforts to discredit the pursuit of enhancements by attributing bad character to those who engage in it, nor attempts to derive prohibitions on enhancement from the concept of human nature or the natural, nor appeals to Conservative insights about humility, spontaneity, and the appreciation of existing goods succeed in establishing the anti-enhancement position—the view that we ought to refrain from enhancements across the board. Nor do any of these objections show that we ought to reject the enhancement enterprise. Further, I've shown that there are weighty reasons in favor of engaging in the enhancement enterprise. I've also argued that it is a mistake to frame the enhancement debate by assuming extreme connectedness among the good and bad features of human beings or between human biology and valuable social relationships. Showing all of that is a far cry, of course, from establishing that any particular enhancement is a good idea or that embarking on the enhancement enterprise is a good idea all things considered. At this point, I have only made a *prima facie* case for cautiously embracing the enhancement enterprise for now—subject to revising the decision in the light of what happens when we begin to engage in it. To make the case for the enhancement enterprise fully convincing, it is necessary to show we could cope with the risks that enhancement would create.

In my judgment, the most serious consideration weighing against the enhancement enterprise is the risk of bad unintended consequences.

How serious the risk will be will depend upon particular features of the proposed enhancement in question and the social circumstances in which it would be used. "Risk" here covers a multitude of potential harms, physical, psychological, and social. In previous chapters, the focus has been on potential psychological and social harms of biomedical enhancement, as well as on moral harms, especially damage to character. In this chapter I concentrate on biological harms: damage to individuals or to the human species that involves loss or impairment of important functionings. More specifically, I want to address the risks of biological harms that could result from what many take to be the most dangerous mode of enhancement: the intentional modification of human germline cells—genetic engineering of embryos or gametes (eggs or sperm)—what I will refer to from now on as IGM (intentional genetic modification).

There are at least three reasons why even those who think that other modes of enhancement are not especially morally problematic may draw the line at IGM. None of them is a good reason.

First, they may think that unintended bad consequences of IGM are more serious than in the case of other modes of biomedical enhancement. Here we need to distinguish between biological harms to the enhanced individual and those to the species. Clearly, the risk of harm to the species is greatly diminished if enhancement by IGM is kept to a very limited scale. It is important to keep this simple point in mind, because sometimes the critics of IGM, including Francis Fukuyama, write as if there is a serious risk that humanity will somehow decide to undergo a massive collective transformation through IGM. Given the expense of IGM, its invasiveness, the cultural and especially religious opposition to it, the well-known attractions of low-tech gene splicing, and the general unruliness of human beings when it comes to reproductive matters, this seems unlikely.

Containment of genetic modifications to the organism in which the alteration is made is not difficult in mammals. It is unlikely, therefore, that an IGM in some humans could inadvertently spread to the wider population. The contrast between IGM in humans and genetic modification of plants is instructive. The most serious risk of unintended harms from the deliberate modification of food crops is that of the unintentional spreading of the alteration. That risk is very low in the case of IGM on humans or other mammals because of the way they reproduce.

Unlike the seeds of genetically modified crops, human gametes are not blown about by the wind; nor do they hitch-hike in the fur of passing animals. The risks of IGM to the individual human will vary depending upon the nature of the genetic alteration. Some other modes of enhancement, such as neural tissue implants or brain–computer interface technologies, may in fact be more risky than some cases of IGM. Even if it is true as a broad generalization that IGM poses greater risk of harm to the individual than other modes of enhancement, if there are enough exceptions and if they can be reliably identified, then the generalization doesn't warrant the conclusion that we should refrain from all IGM, much less that it should be banned as a matter of public policy. Later, I'll introduce cautionary heuristics, based on the evolutionary biology of ontogeny— the development of an organism from the individual to maturity. These heuristics provide a more fine-grained approach to risk assessment than such clumsy generalizations as "IGM is more risky than other modes of enhancement." Here I simply want to stress that in assessing the risks of IGM, it is crucial to avoid gene fetishism: the mere fact that a change is a genetic one does not make it a major change. It all depends on the gene or genes in question. Some nongenetic biomedical enhancements, such as neural tissue implants or even the administration of mood-altering drugs, may have much greater effects than many genetic modifications.

Second, some may try to draw a bright line that excludes any IGM because they mistakenly assume that if such interventions produced unintended bad consequences, they would be irreversible. That, too, is a mistake—one which confuses genotype with phenotype. Whether a genetic change produces a change in phenotype depends on the complex regulatory functions that determine whether the gene is activated, as well as the environment in which it is expressed. Scientists already know how to block the expression of genes they insert into laboratory animals. They can modify the inserted gene so that it will not be expressed unless deliberately activated by the administration of a drug, and they can block the expression of inserted genes by the administration of a drug.

Third, blanket opposition to IGM may rest on the assumption that it, unlike other modes of biomedical enhancement, "changes our biology" and that this makes it more dangerous. I have already indicated why this way of framing the issue is misleading: some genetic modifications will be rather limited in their effects, so it would be misleading to say they have changed our biology.

More importantly, whether changing our biology could in some circumstances be a good thing obviously depends on what our biology is like, and our best information about what it is like comes from medical science that is informed by evolutionary biology. So my strategy in this chapter will be to try to determine, on the basis of an understanding of some basic points of that science, whether it is correct to assume that we should not change our biology.

Before proceeding, I want to make it clear that I, like many other bioethicists, think that the single most important obstacle to the ethically permissible use of IGM in humans is the problem of figuring out how to conduct ethical research on IGM with humans. As I noted in Chapter One, I am not going to address that issue directly in this volume. Instead, I'll proceed hypothetically, asking how we should evaluate the biological risks of IGM, on the assumption that we have devised a way of conducting ethical research designed to develop this mode of enhancement. Nevertheless, much of what I say about risk reduction will be significant for the problem of IGM research ethics. In particular, the cautionary heuristics I set out later in this chapter could play a central role in determining which lines of research are sufficiently safe to be ethically permissible.

Costs and *benefits*

When applied to the problem of the risk of unintended biological harms, the upshot of my argument in previous chapters is this: we should dispose of faulty analogies and dubious assumptions about extreme connectedness, and try to weigh the risks against benefits of particular enhancements in the light of the best scientific information we have. The anti-enhancement writers I have criticized in preceding chapters disagree. They declare that to focus on bad unintended consequences is superficial and they scorn what they see as the tendency to reduce the complexities of the enhancement debate to a calculation of costs and benefits.[1]

Cost–benefit analysis, strictly understood, is a valuable tool that can contribute to the evaluation of actions and policies, but its usefulness is quite limited. For one thing, it requires that all costs and benefits be quantifiable by a common measure (e.g., dollars) and in some important cases this is not feasible. For another, cost–benefit analysis, as it is often used, is completely insensitive to considerations of fairness, deserts, and entitlement. It only addresses the balance of benefits over costs, not the distribution of either. These limitations of cost–benefit analysis are now universally acknowledged among those who advocate its use. If Sandel's criticism is directed against those who think that cost–benefit analysis, strictly speaking, can resolve issues in the ethics of enhancement, he is attacking a strawman.

Sometimes, talk of costs and benefits does not imply a commitment to using cost–benefit analysis. Instead, as I have emphasized in earlier chapters, it is equivalent to talk about pros and cons. In this broader, less formal sense, looking at costs and benefits is commonsensical—a matter of trying to articulate the full range of considerations that count in favor of or against a course of action or a policy, and then attempting to make an all-things-considered judgment about what to do. There is no assumption that the pros and cons can be neatly quantified and rendered commensurate. Thinking about costs and benefits in this way does not give short shrift to considerations of character or of the quality of human relationships. On the contrary, an appropriate consideration of costs in the broadest sense requires us to take these matters into account. It also can accommodate the equally commonsensical idea that there is more than one value to be taken into account in making decisions about enhancement, and that the mere fact that the pursuit of enhancement *might* worsen bad character traits or is *sometimes* the expression of bad character is not a sufficient reason to refrain from it, if it serves other important values, such as improving human well-being.

Ironically, those who deprecate the alleged shallowness of the concern with consequences invariably appeal to consequences themselves. As we saw in Chapter Three, Sandel predicts that the availability of enhancements will exacerbate character flaws that already exist. Similarly, we saw in Chapter Four that the President's Council predicts that a society in which genetic engineering of embryos for enhancement is widespread will be one in which procreation comes to be (or at least to be seen as) a kind of manufacturing. These are predictions of bad consequences. As such, they require empirical support, though those who make them fail to provide it. Just as importantly, these predictions are apparently offered as conclusive reasons for refraining from enhancement. But that is a mistake, because it overlooks the possibility that the risk of bad consequences might be outweighed by the benefits of enhancement, or by a combination of the benefits of enhancement and the value of liberty, both scientific and personal. Merely pointing out a speculative risk of some bad consequence is not enough to make an "argument against enhancement."

The difficult route from the identification of a risk associated with doing X to the conclusion that we ought not to do X has four main stages, *all* of which are blithely omitted by writers like Sandel, Kass, Annas, and Habermas. The first is to try to determine not only the magnitude of the possible harm, but also the probability of its occurrence. The second, which I have already noted, is to consider the full range of possible benefits of doing X (not just the least respectable ones) and to determine how probable they are. The third is to determine whether there are morally acceptable, affordable, and effective risk-prevention or risk-reduction measures that would allow us to reap the benefits of doing X without running an unacceptable risk of bad consequences. Notice the qualifier "unacceptable." In the real world, the elimination of risk is virtually impossible and not acting can be as risky, or riskier, than acting .

One cannot merely cite risks and omit any consideration of possible offsetting benefits, unless one has good reason to believe that the risks are so serious as to exclude any consideration of benefits. None of the anti-enhancement arguments examined so far comes close to doing this. It is as if their proponents had registered for a course on risk–benefit analysis and dropped out before the concept of benefits was introduced. To make matters worse, to the extent that the harshest critics of enhancement consider possible benefits at all, they do so in an extremely one-sided and prejudicial way by focusing exclusively on competitive advantage, vanity, or the indulgence of wild-eyed desires for mastery or perfection. (Recall Sandel's not so subtle bait and switch: the title of his book is *The Case Against Perfection* and his only cogent arguments are against the pursuit of perfection, but he claims to be providing an "argument against enhancement."[2] The point is that seeking to improve is not the same as seeking perfection.)

I've exposed these errors by showing that some of the most widely discussed biomedical enhancements may bring genuinely valuable benefits (and not just to those who have the enhancements) and may be pursued for respectable, even admirable, reasons. I have also argued that some of the risks that the critics of enhancement identify are not really risks at all. In particular, since there is nothing wrong *per se* with changing human nature, the possibility that enhancement will change human nature is not in itself a risk, much less an unacceptable risk, as I argued in Chapter Four.

In the rest of this chapter, I address the problem of unintended bad consequences in its most tangible form—the risk of biological harms. Before doing so, I want to probe the claim, advanced by some prominent anti-enhancement writers, that there is something superficial— dangerously superficial—about thinking in terms of costs (or risks) *and benefits*.

There are two distinct reasons why critics of enhancement might think that any consideration of costs and benefits reveals a kind of moral shallowness. Their point might be that only a moral simpleton would think that all pros and cons can be neatly quantified in the way cost–benefit analysis (strictly speaking) requires. I have already noted that this criticism is aimed at a strawman, since virtually no one in the enhancement debate has suggested that the issues can be resolved by cost–benefit analysis in the strict sense. Alternatively, their point might be that there are some risks that are so morally momentous that it is inappropriate even to consider whether any benefits could outweigh them—that a proper appreciation of the nature of some risks should put a stop to the process of weighing pros and cons.

It is true that some risks may sometimes count as conclusive— considerations that rule out taking countervailing considerations into account or that at least create a presumption that they are not to be considered. In Chapter Two, I considered the possibility that Sandel and Habermas think that they have identified conclusive reasons against enhancement. I then argued that none of the worries about enhancement they raise is a good candidate for being a conclusive reason. Habermas's concern that a child who grew from an embryo whose genotype was designed could not regard herself as free is based on either a genetic determinist confusion (between designing the genotype of an embryo and designing a child) or on a muddled conception of what makes an individual free (the mistake of thinking that it is her origins rather than her characteristics). Sandel's warnings about hyper-parenting and his unseemly attempt to discredit the motivation of everyone who seeks enhancement by portraying them as perfectionists or mastery freaks fall far short of constituting reasons to rule out all consideration of the benefits of enhancement.

So far, then, we have no reason to believe that there are conclusive reasons against biomedical enhancement and hence no reason not to pursue the commonsense strategy of looking at costs ("cons") *and* benefits ("pros") and trying to come to an all-things-considered judgment that gives us guidance as to what to do. Nonetheless, in what follows I do not assume that there are no such conclusive reasons. Instead, my strategy is to avoid prejudging the issue. In earlier chapters I have articulated possible benefits of enhancement and did something to show that some of them—especially cognitive enhancements—appear to have a significant probability of being realized, given the history of previous, nonbiomedical enhancements. In this chapter I consider the problem of risks, at the outset leaving open the possibility that we will determine that the risks of IGM are so great that we should ban this mode of enhancement, in spite of its benefits. The point is that it is one thing to conclude, *after* an impartial investigation, that the risks outweigh the benefits; it is quite another to assume that certain risks preclude any attempt to determine whether the risks outweigh the benefits.

The problem of unintended bad consequences is so serious and so complex that it would take more than a whole volume to begin to address it in a convincing way. My aim in this chapter is more modest. I want to *begin* the task of thinking responsibly about the risk that biomedical enhancement efforts will produce bad unintended consequences by focusing on unintended biological harms that might be caused by IGM, the most controversial type of biomedical enhancement. Here as elsewhere, my emphasis will be on how to frame the issue properly, and this will involve clearing away a good deal of rubbish before the foundations for fruitful thinking can be constructed.

Many consider IGM to be the most risky mode of enhancement. If I can make a convincing case that under realistic circumstances IGM would in some cases be permissible, then I will have shown that it is wrong to try to draw a bright line that excludes biomedical enhancements generally as being too risky. A more constructive aim of the chapter is to help remedy one of the defects in the thinking of those who have *not* recommended complete abstinence from IGM. As I noted in Chapter One, writers who reject the view that we should never engage in biomedical enhancement uniformly recognize that the risk of unintended bad consequences is a serious problem. But they typically say too little about how we are to cope with this problem, resting content with remarks about the importance of "going slow" and "proceeding with caution." I aim to do better than that.

Alternative Strategies for Coping With Risk

I begin by contrasting three fundamentally different approaches to the risk of unintended bad biological consequences of IGM: (1) prohibition of the risky behavior, (2) reliance on a single, master risk-reducing principle, such as the Precautionary Principle, or (3) employing a plurality of cautionary heuristics that are sensitive to changes in our knowledge about risk *and* that encourage us to gain more knowledge that is relevant to assessing risk. Each will be considered in turn. My conclusion will be that the third alternative is superior.

Prohibition

Applied to the case of IGM, the prohibition strategy means drawing a bright line (or erecting a moral firebreak) between enhancements that involve IGM and those that do not, and strictly prohibiting the former. There are two quite different rationales for this prohibition strategy. The first is to base it on the view that IGM for any purpose is wrong in every instance, while other modes of enhancement may sometimes be permissible. This first rationale is hard to defend, at least if one concedes that in some cases IGM may have permissible therapeutic uses. If a lethal disease could only be prevented by genetically modifying gametes (for example, through testicular vaccination) or gene surgery on embryos, then presumably this would be permissible.

Alternatively, one might hold that *therapeutic* IGM is sometimes permissible but *enhancement* IGM never is, either by arguing (1) that there is something wrong with enhancement *per se* (for example, that it is always motivated by unseemly desires for perfection or because it is contrary to our nature) or (2) that enhancement IGM always carries greater risks than therapeutic IGM. Neither alternative is attractive: enhancement is not wrong *per se* (as I have argued in the preceding chapters), and some IGM enhancements may be much less risky than some IGM treatments; it will all depend upon the nature of the genetic change that is made.

One needn't hold such implausible views as (1) and (2) to find the idea of a bright line attractive, however. One might concede that there are some cases in which IGM enhancement would be morally permissible, but that the most responsible course of action is to avoid all IGM enhancements nonetheless. One could argue that we are too prone to error in judging whether a particular IGM enhancement would be a good idea. The bright line prohibition strategy on this second rationale serves as a kind of cognitive self-binding device: we avoid errors of judgment by taking the opportunity to commit them off the table. On the second rationale, the distinction is valuable as an epistemic proxy: we judge better if we treat the distinction *as if* it were of moral significance than if we try to ascertain the moral permissibility of enhancement case by case.

Whether the epistemic proxy rationale provides an adequate grounding for the prohibition of enhancement IGM depends upon two factors: how prone we are to underestimate the risk in particular instances of enhancement IGM *and* how great the potential benefits of enhancement IGM are (what the opportunity costs of following the prohibition strategy are). In the next two sections, I address both of these factors. IGM is to be contrasted with UGM—unintentional genetic modification, the germline modifications that occur through evolution without deliberate human intervention in the germline. In "IGM versus UGM or a critical look at the wisdom of nature" I argue that because of the limitations of UGM as a mechanism for preserving and promoting human well-being, and the potential of IGM to overcome these limitations, the opportunity costs of forgoing IGM are very high. (The opportunity cost of doing X is the value of the most valuable foregone alternative.) In "A better way to think responsibly about intentional genetic modification," I argue for a set of cautionary heuristics that are a more reasonable response to the problem of risk than a blanket prohibition on enhancement IGM. I show that, given our current state of knowledge and, more importantly, the fact that our knowledge is growing, there are better ways to cope with error in judgments about the risks of IGM than by a blanket prohibition on it.

IGM Versus UGM or A Critical Look at the Wisdom of Nature[3]

The history of life has only very recently produced a species whose understanding of evolution makes possible the *intentional* modification of its own genome. As I have already noted, we already have considerable knowledge of the biological effects of specific genetic modifications in laboratory animals with respect to genes they share with humans and of the effects of specific genetic variations in humans. There is mounting evidence that human beings will eventually be able to change their physical, cognitive, and emotional capacities by modifying their genes.[4]

Advocates of a prohibition on IGM often declare that it is foolish to disregard the wisdom of nature. Some who make this charge explicitly appeal to science rather than religion: they explicate the idea of the wisdom of nature by recourse to the Master Engineer Analogy already encountered in Chapter Five's examination of the implications of Conservative thought for enhancement. They believe that from an evolutionary perspective, the human organism is like the product of an engineering genius—a "delicately balanced," completed, well-functioning masterwork. On this view, IGM is likely to be disastrously counterproductive, like the blundering efforts of a child to improve on the intricate, well-thought-out work of an engineering genius. Recall the stern warning issued by the (US) President's Council on Bioethics:

> The human body and mind, highly complex and delicately balanced as the result of eons of gradual and exacting evolution, are almost certainly at risk from any ill-considered attempt at "improvement".... It is far from clear that our delicately integrated natural bodily powers will take kindly to such impositions, however desirable the sought-for change may seem to the intervener.[5]

Notice that if the Master Engineer analogy is apt, there is at least a strong presumption against IGM for any reason whatsoever, not just for purposes of enhancement. If evolution is a like a Master Engineer and we are like clumsy, ignorant children, then it is too dangerous to try to alter the Master Engineer's products, whether human or otherwise, even to prevent disease or avert some ecological catastrophe of our own making.

The Master Engineer analogy, as I argued in Chapter Five, has two close relatives: the House of Cards and Seamless Web analogies. The unifying idea behind all three analogies is that of *extreme connectedness.*

What matters, ultimately, is the assumption of extreme connectedness, not the analogies used to convey it. Drawing on well-established findings from evolutionary biology, I argued in Chapter Five that human beings and other evolved beings are *not* characterized by the extreme connectedness conveyed by these analogies. In particular, canalization, modularity, and redundancy are pervasive biological phenomena that limit connectedness and thereby reduce the risk that either human interventions or environmental changes or mutations will seriously disrupt the functioning of organisms. I also pointed out that from the standpoint of natural selection, one would not expect extreme connectedness, because organisms that exhibited it would tend to be weeded out because of their fragility.

There are two fundamental problems for appeals to extreme connectedness as a *conclusive* reason against human interventions into biological systems or individual organisms. The first and most damaging is that the assumption of extreme connectedness is a dubious dogma. Of course, there are connections, within and across organisms, but from this it does not follow that every intervention is likely to produce unacceptable disruptions of benign dependencies. The second problem is that if the extreme connectedness assumption were valid, it is likely that human action has *already* produced such serious disruptions that further interventions may well be needed to correct for them. In other words, if nature is as fragile as the extreme connectedness assumption implies, what reason do we have to think that it can recover from the disruptions we have already wrought on it? On the other hand, if it is resilient enough to recover without our help, this means that it is not as fragile as the extreme connectedness assumption says it is. My focus, however, is on the first problem: the lack of empirical support for the extreme connectedness assumption.

Human beings, like all organisms, are fragile in the sense that their survival depends on continued adaption to a changing environment—as the Red Queen Hypothesis has it, organisms have to run ever faster as the ground crumbles beneath their feet. They are also fragile in the sense that the predictable "endpoint" of evolution is the dustbin of extinction (not the pinnacle of progress). But these sorts of fragility are compatible with the limitations on connectedness that result from canalization, modularity, and redundancy. The more we learn about the biology of human beings, the greater our prospects for intervening without unacceptable risk of disrupting benign dependencies. And as I argued in Chapters Two and Five, we may need to intervene in order to avert various harms—from pandemics to global warming to carcinogens in the water we drink to sharp declines in fertility due to environmental toxins—including those we have produced. Given what we *already* know, the extreme connectedness assumption is incapable of grounding a ban on biomedical enhancement generally or on enhancement utilizing IGM in particular. Germline modifications of laboratory animals have already produced significant phenotypic changes without a catastrophic unraveling of the Seamless Web or a collapse of the House of Cards. My point is *not* that we should replace the extreme connectedness assumption with an equally unfounded assumption of extreme unconnectedness. Rather, we should avoid *a priorism* in either direction, steer clear of sweeping generalizations, and look at the facts in all their particularity. Unfortunately, the metaphors that opponents of IGM use divert our attention from the facts that are relevant to assessing the risk of this mode of enhancement.

The constraints of UGM

If Darwinian theory effectively banished intelligent design from evolutionary explanation,[6] what could philosophers mean when they attribute "wisdom" to nature and then appeal to it as a reason against IGM? Their idea is that over eons of evolutionary trial and error, the Darwinian crucible has produced ingenious solutions to challenging design problems, achieving a degree of perfection that humans are overwhelmingly unlikely to improve upon. According to this view, which we encountered in Chapter Five, organisms (including human beings) are like the finished products of a Master Engineer.

Even scientifically sophisticated bioethicists with a generally positive view of IGM have a tendency to rely on the Master Engineer analogy when they address the problem of unintended bad consequences. For instance, Bostrom and Sandberg caution that when "an over-ambitious tinkerer with merely superficial understanding of what he is doing [makes] changes to the design of a Master Engineer, the potential for damage is considerable and the chances of producing an all-things-considered improvement are small."[7]

But as I argued in Chapter Five, organisms are remarkably *unlike* the work of a Master Engineer in two fundamental respects. First, unlike a Master Engineer, evolution never gets the job done: organisms are not the endpoints of an evolutionary process that gradually but steadily climbs the ladder of perfection. The ladder is always being pulled out from under the organism—the environment is ever-changing and adaptations are one step behind. Hence organisms are not delicately balanced finished products in danger of being upset or destroyed by human intervention. Second, evolution does not "design" what it produces according to a plan that exists (even if only in rough outline) at the beginning of production. Each of these points and their significance for the Master Engineer analogy will become clear as we carefully consider the constraints under which UGM operates. Once the severity of these constraints is appreciated, it becomes clear that the Master Engineer analogy is incapable of supporting a prohibition on or even a strong presumption against IGM. On the contrary, the fact that IGM has the potential to overcome these powerful constraints on UGM provides a strong case for developing the capacity to employ it.

Broadly speaking, "constraints" in evolutionary biology refer to circumstances limiting the nature of design problems and their set of possible solutions. Here I use the term differently. The evolutionary features listed below, some of which we already encountered in Chapter Five, are constraints in the sense of limitations on the effectiveness of UGM—unassisted evolution—*as a process by which to promote (or even preserve) human well-being.*

1. The ubiquity of suboptimal design
It is ironic that proponents of the Master Engineer analogy regard the theory of natural selection as the basis for the analogy, since it is the *imperfection* of biological design that is among the strongest evidence for evolution by natural selection. Darwin himself frequently pointed to the faulty, irrational construction of organisms in the service of rebuking arguments for intentional (and intelligent) design.

There is no need to repeat the long list of suboptimal design features of humans offered in Chapter Five. The point is that the ubiquity of suboptimal design demonstrates that natural selection is a *bricoleur*, not an engineer, much less a Master Engineer—that is, it tinkers with organisms in response to immediate need, co-opting existing structures in *ad hoc* fashion to meet new functional demands. When we consider the *mechanisms* (2–10 below) that originate and maintain suboptimal engineering in nature, it becomes clear why less-than-masterful design is not the exception but rather the rule for UGM.

2. Selection is insensitive to the postreproductive quality of life

Beyond a certain age, organisms contribute little to the gene pool of the next generation, and thus with some rare and controversial exceptions, natural selection tends not to act on the postreproductive period of life. This simple truth has enormous implications for the Master Engineer analogy, for if natural selection is the sole driver of optimality, then the vast majority of postreproductive traits do not benefit from evolution's putative engineering genius. Therefore, the notion that all or even most biological traits are the direct result or necessary side-effect of natural selection is patently false. Once its reproductive years are over, organisms are allowed to "drift," with selection no longer investing in the physiological repair mechanisms necessary to prevent the accumulation of mutations in cell lines that can lead to cancer, cardiovascular disease, and neural degeneration. This dynamic is of particular relevance in the case of long-lived organisms like humans, who (at least nowadays) spend substantial fractions of their life in the postreproductive period.

One of the chief advantages of IGM is that it can avoid or ameliorate the harms that humans suffer as a result of UGM's insensitivity to their postreproductive quality of life. For example, modifications of oncogenes or tumor-suppressing genes could reduce the incidence of cancer in later life,[8] and changes in the genetic networks that regulate hormones could prevent or retard muscle loss and frailty in elderly people.[9]

3. Selection, optimality and improvement

The Master Engineer analogy hinges on three chief assumptions: (1) selection is the predominant mechanism determining biological traits; (2) selection tends to produce traits that are optimal; and (3) optimal traits cannot be improved upon by IGM. All of these assumptions are dubious. There is good reason to doubt (1): recent work in the philosophy of biology has shown that drift is actually the default state of biological systems.[10] But even if selection did overwhelm all other evolutionary tendencies and constraints, this would not imply that any trait produced by natural selection is optimal. Recall that "adaptation" (in the most uncontroversial sense) refers to the *etiology* of a trait—in particular, the fact that it *arose* and *came* to fixation (with emphasis on the past tense) as a result of natural selection. By contrast, "optimality" refers to the *current* function of a trait and its present contribution to reproductive fitness irrespective of its selective history.[11] This distinction is important, as we cannot assume that the same forces that originally selected for a trait are the ones that currently maintain it. A trait that evolved for some purpose in the distant past may persist long after that initial design problem is gone, due either to a shift in its function ("exaptation") or to various evolutionary impediments to extinguishing it.

Even if selection was the sole significant evolutionary mechanism, and even if it did produce traits that were optimal, this would still not imply (3). Simply because a trait has been optimized by natural selection does not mean that it cannot be improved upon. To conflate "optimal" with "un-improvable" is to misunderstand the concept of optimality as it is used in evolutionary theory. Although the link between adaptation and optimality remains empirically and conceptually tenuous,[12] this much is clear: any optimality analysis will be relative to certain genetic, developmental, and functional parameters. Abstracted from these engineering constraints, the concept of optimality becomes unintelligible.[13] In essence, to say that a trait is optimal is to say that no further *incremental* changes in the genotype can improve on the function of the trait. This is consistent with the notion that *nonincremental* changes could transport a lineage to a higher fitness peak in the overall adaptive landscape (see discussion below). I will say more about the advantages of nonincremental genetic modification shortly. For now, it is enough to recognize that given the local nature of biological optimality, we should view IGM as expanding the range of the developmentally possible, rather than threatening a masterpiece of selection.[14]

In addition, the degree of optimality that can be achieved in nature is highly constrained by the topography of the "adaptive landscape." This latter phrase refers to a pictorial representation of the functional relationship between individual genotype/phenotypes and the environment. If the landscape comprises numerous fitness peaks and valleys, then selection will cause a population to climb the nearest fitness peak, even if that peak is not the highest one in the landscape. It will henceforth be stranded on this globally suboptimal peak, since to navigate to a higher one would entail that it cross a region of low fitness, which stabilizing selection will not permit ("stabilizing selection" is selection that favors the mean phenotype, while weeding out values on the tail ends of the phenotypic distribution). In such cases, adaptive suboptimality persists because of—not despite—natural selection. What appears to be an optimal solution from a local vantage point may be highly suboptimal when viewed panoramically—a perspective that is well beyond the ken of UGM. With a bird's eye view of the adaptive landscape, however, IGM could prevent a population from being locked into a local optimum by identifying the highest peak, circumventing spatiotemporal barriers to gene flow, and coordinating the non-incremental assembly and dissemination of complex adaptations from the genes of disparate populations.

Not only is optimality inherently local and context-dependent, it may not even correlate with long-term species survival. Thus, contrary to the Master Engineer analogy, existing traits (including our own) do not represent the adaptive apex of eons of exacting selection; rather, they are ecologically provisional, may not be ideally suited for their current function, and are not necessarily superior in design to those that litter the fossil beds.

4. Evolutionary "hangovers"

To say that a trait is an adaptation is to say that it is the product of a historical selective regime. As was just noted, since the environment and the design problems it poses are constantly in flux, organisms can never be perfectly adapted to their environment. Thus, many of the traits that were fitness-conferring in early hominid evolution may be either neutral or maladaptive today. Such likely "Pleistocene hangovers" range from the predilection toward sweet, salty, and fatty foods, to stepchild abuse and xenophobia.[15] Evolutionary psychologists believe that many of our contemporary psychological disorders, such as depression, anxiety, and attention deficit disorder, stem from difficulties associated with the psychological transition from hunter-gathering to a more sedentary, agriculture-based existence. A similar diagnosis applies to many of the disorders observed in canine companion animals, who with equal difficulty are forced to adjust from a roaming pack life to the confines of the living room sofa.

5. The origination and fixation of mutations

Another obvious limitation on UGM as a means of improving or sustaining human well-being is the *manner* in which beneficial mutations originate and spread, a process that can take thousands or even millions of years, depending on mutation rates, population structure, and the type of the adaptation in question. While strong selection pressures may speed up genetic evolution, they also entail the lamentable Malthusian scenario in which there are far more births than environmental resources can support. For instance, ancestral human populations had to sustain enormous death rates from small pox and bubonic plague in order to achieve widespread pathogen resistance.[16] The end result may be agreeable, but the process leading up to it can be nasty, brutish, and long. IGM has the potential to achieve equally good results without the horrific costs.

For example, suppose we learn that some desirable gene or complex of genes already exists, but only in a small number of humans (this has proved to be the case, for example, with respect to resistance to certain strains of HIV). Waiting for this genotype to spread through the human population at UGM's usual measured pace would be not only statistically problematic (given the potential for the variant to be eliminated by drift), but also morally catastrophic. An unrelated epidemic, armed conflict, or some other chance event could destroy the critical population of humans; and even if no such event occurred, fixation might take thousands of years, during which time millions of people who lacked the genotype would die or suffer serious illness. Suppose also that it were possible to ensure the much more rapid proliferation of the genotype by administering an injection into the testes or, more radically, by inserting genes into embryos in the context of *in vitro* fertilization. In this way, IGM could not only realize the same beneficial outcome that UGM is capable of achieving, but it could do so much more reliably, quickly, and with far less human carnage. From a moral perspective, this should count heavily in favor of IGM. In addition, because it is not subject to the vagaries of un-assisted evolution, IGM technology can safeguard valuable genotypes much as early humans cradled fire, protecting the genetic resources needed for survival for current and future generations.

6. The improbability of "lateral" gene transfer in the UGM of animals.

Microbes have the evolutionary upper hand when it comes to the arms race between simple parasites and their complex animal hosts. The transmission of desirable mutations in complex multicellular animals is laborious, given long generation times and the fact that reproduction and gene transfer are inextricably linked. This is in stark contrast to bacterial life forms, which have both rapid generation times and "lateral" modes of gene transfer. Lateral transmission enables simple organisms to exchange genes outside of sexual reproduction, allowing for the more efficient proliferation of fitness-enhancing traits. IGM can act in complex multi-cellular species as lateral gene transfer does in prokaryotes, greatly increasing the speed and versatility with which salutary mutations can spread through the population. IGM allows us to combine and integrate the genes of human beings who are not members of the same lineage, as well as genes from other species and those artificially created via synthetic biology. Like cultural exchange between unrelated members of a population, lateral gene transfer comes with attendant risks, including the more rapid spread of deleterious variants that would otherwise be contained to vertical lineages. Nevertheless, IGM promises to even the evolutionary arms race between the agile parasites and the lumbering human populations they track.

7. Linkage, epistasis, and macromutation

The blind and incremental nature of natural selection not only places severe constraints on how quickly natural selection can accomplish a given adaptive feat, but also on which adaptive feats can be accomplished at all. Mutation and recombination, which together provide the raw materials for natural selection in sexual organisms, impose severe constraints on what selection has to work with and how it can do so. For example, consider the ubiquitous phenomenon known as "linkage disequilibrium": when fitness-enhancing genes are located on the chromosome close to neutral or maladaptive genes, they will be bound together in the recombinatory shuffle and jointly destined to enter the next generation, despite the maladaptive genes' detrimental effect on the phenotype. This assumes, of course, that the net gain in fitness associated with the beneficial gene outweighs the net cost from its being linked to a deleterious gene. If the benefits do not outweigh the costs of linkage, then selection will be unable to favor (i.e., differentially produce) the salutary variant. Similar limitations arise from "pleiotropism," where single genes code for multiple unrelated functions, and "epistatic interactions," in which the developmental state of one gene affects the function of another.

Furthermore, because natural selection is an *incremental* process, it faces insurmountable hurdles when confronted with a design problem that requires hundreds or even thousands of *simultaneous* mutations to solve. Consider a scenario in which the individually necessary and jointly sufficient mutations for some beneficial trait fail to confer a fitness benefit either individually or in any combination other than the final one. The probability of realizing any particular mutational trajectory is equal to the product of the probabilities of its constituent mutations. As the number of requisite mutations grows, the chance they will be realized simultaneously or in the right order decreases exponentially. By contrast, what is an astronomically improbable feat for natural selection can be a relatively simple task for a human engineer. Macromutations are well within the forward-looking, goal-oriented ambit of IGM.

Thus, not only can IGM usher in sweeping genetic change at a much faster pace than UGM, but it has access to entire regions of adaptive space that are off limits to natural selection. In this way, IGM could be an invaluable resource—literally a matter of life or death for the species—in the case where humans are confronted with an imminent design problem, the solution to which is either totally inaccessible to incremental selection, or else only achievable over vast stretches of evolutionary time. For example, IGM might enable us to alter the body's capacity for thermal regulation in response to global warming, or increase our resistance to emerging pathogens or our tolerance of environmental toxicity. In theory, by tapping into the master regulatory pathways of developing organisms, IGM has the potential to go well beyond trait *enhancement* to the wholesale *transformation* of biological organization.

8. Optimization of one trait is not improvement overall

Because of the integrated nature of organisms, even if one trait is "optimized" by natural selection, this does not preclude it from having detrimental consequences for other traits, so long as the fitness benefit associated with the former is strong enough to compensate for the damage done to the latter. For instance, in early hominid evolution, there was strong selection for bipedalism, likely due to the scattering of resources and the inefficiency of knuckle-walking as a mode of transport. Apparently, the fitness benefits from bipedalism were so great that they outweighed the substantial costs associated with the hasty reconstruction of hominid anatomy in order to accommodate this new form of loco-motion. The costs of this highly constrained evolutionary tradeoff include some of the highest rates of neonatal and maternal mortality in the animal kingdom, not to mention a host of debilitating knee and back problems. On top of this, human medical technology has greatly reduced the incidence of child mortality (via, for example, Caesarean section), relaxing any selection pressures for additional beneficial mod-ifications of the pelvis. Even when medical technology can compensate for biological suboptimality, however, this does not mean that IGM is unnecessary or unwarranted, especially given that complex cultural solutions may often come at a much higher social price than a basic genetic fix.

9. Species extinction and the irrevocable loss of genes.

When species become extinct in nature, their distinctive genes are usually lost forever. In contrast, human-initiated gene banks (akin to the Global Seed Vault, which recently opened in Norway) can be maintained long after extinction in the wild, and genetic information can even be resurrected from fossil materials. Such stored or recovered genes could be reinserted in the human germline as needed. In this way, IGM can stave off and even reverse extinction events that would other-wise be inevitable or irrevocable. Ironically, then, the common criticism that IGM ought to be banned because it might result in irreparable loss of potentially valuable genetic material applies with even greater force to UGM.

10. The most profound constraint of all: UGM selects for fitness, not human good

To say that a trait increases reproductive fitness is just to say that it increases the probability that the genes of the organism bearing the trait will be passed on to future generations, either through the organism's own reproduction or through that of its kin. Even if every human trait contributed to reproductive fitness (not true), and even if any

IGM-based change would be likely to reduce overall fitness (also not true), it would *still* not follow that any effort to improve humans via IGM is likely to make humans *worse off*, for the simple reason that human well-being is not the same as reproductive fitness. If we plot the desirability of traits against their contribution to inclusive fitness, there may be significant overlap between the curves, but they will not perfectly map onto one another. This is because maximizing the number of genes the current generation passes on is not the only thing of value, if it is of value at all, either for individual humans or for humanity collectively.

It might turn out, for example, that to maximize the number of genes the current generation passes on, the best strategy would be to increase the human population up to the Malthusian breaking point—that is, to have as many offspring as possible, even if this meant that all the survivors should be merely subsisting in conditions of dire poverty, deprived of most of what makes for a good human life. The point is that fitness only concerns the expected *number* of viable offspring—it remains totally insensitive to either the parent or the offspring's *quality of life*. One person's conception of the good may be to have as many offspring as they can in their short time on Earth; for others, having fewer (or no) offspring enables them to pursue other sorts of projects that make their life meaningful; and yet still others may choose to forgo reproduction altogether in order to adopt unrelated children who are in need of care.

Dawkins's famous blind watchmaker analogy obscures the most profound constraint on UGM—namely, its effectiveness as a means of achieving human good—because it encourages a fundamentally mistaken view of what natural selection is about. It is not about human improvement. When UGM, operating through natural selection, produces what is valuable for human beings, it does so by sheer coincidence. It would be unwise to wager the prospects of human survival, much less the prospects for improvement, on sheer coincidence.

A better analogy would be this: UGM is like the work of a morally blind, fickle, and tightly shackled tinkerer. The tinkerer is *morally blind* in a two-fold sense: he does not have human well-being as a goal and he shows no scruples in his choice of means for achieving his ends. If a (transient) adaptation is achievable only by massive death and suffering, that is no concern of his. He is a *tinkerer*, not a Master Engineer, because he does not produce objects according to a plan conceived in advance;

furthermore, he is fickle in that he always destroys his handiwork eventually, often before he has achieved his extraordinarily limited goals (i.e., producing solutions to immediate design problems without regard to long-term consequences). He is *tightly shackled* in the sense that he operates under severe constraints—potentially useful tools lie all about him, but he cannot reach them because he is tethered in a small corner of a vast workshop. The proposal to intervene in the work of a morally blind, tightly shackled tinkerer looks far more promising than the proposal to modify the work of a Master Engineer.

The limitations of analogies

By this stage of the argument, perhaps we should be wary of all analogies. The Master Engineer, House of Cards, and Seamless Web analogies are misleading because they obscure crucial facts of evolution, facts that are directly relevant to our efforts to assess the risks of enhancement. The analogy of evolution as a blind, morally insensitive, fickle, tightly shackled tinkerer has some value, at least as an antidote to the rosy, pre-Darwinian, teleological view of evolved organisms as harmonious, stable, well-designed, and complete. Once its work of debunking the Master Engineer analogy is done, however, it is not clear how much light this darkly Darwinian analogy can shed on issues of enhancement. The wiser course seems to be to avoid reliance on analogies altogether, make our assessment of the risks of biomedical enhancements on the basis of the best scientific information we have, and then, if the benefits of enhancement are sufficiently valuable, development risk-reduction strategies that are equally scientifically informed.

A Better Way to Think Responsibly about Intentional Genetic Modification

Thus far, I have argued that once the inadequacy of UGM as a process for sustaining or promoting human well-being is appreciated, and once the profligate moral costs of the process are duly considered, the prospect of IGM looks more favorable. For IGM has the potential to overcome the severe constraints under which UGM operates, and can be used in such a way as to reduce or avoid the death and suffering that results from whatever improvement in the human condition UGM might happen to achieve.

I have *not* argued that IGM poses no serious risks. Indeed, everything said so far is compatible with the conclusion that IGM in humans ought not to be undertaken. I now want to suggest that instead of appealing to the wisdom of nature or the genius of the Master Engineer of evolution, it would be better to focus more directly on the risk that intentional genetic modifications (like other human actions) can have unintended bad consequences, and then develop strategies for attempting to reduce this risk. Framing the matter of due caution regarding IGM as a matter of risk *reduction* is appropriate, given the fact that IGM has the potential to promote human good more effectively and at lower moral cost than UGM. Given the good that might be attained by and *only* by IGM, some risk may be worth bearing.

The inadequacy of adaptationist cautionary heuristics

I noted earlier that Bostrom and Sandberg, two philosophers who reject any prohibition or strong presumption against IGM, nonetheless take the Master Engineer analogy seriously and assume that it provides a sound basis for caution about the use of IGM. To their credit, instead of resting content with the platitude that we should "go slow" or "proceed with caution" in the use of IGM, these philosophers go on to offer a set of contentful cautionary heuristics, based, as they see it, on an apprecia-tion of evolutionary theory. The difficulty is that their view of evolution, and hence their cautionary heuristics, is colored by an increasingly discredited understanding of evolution—namely, "strong adaptation-ism," a view which presupposes the inexorable tendency of natural selection to overcome developmental constraints that would otherwise lead to adaptive suboptimality.[17] But even if this were the correct view of evolution, Bostrom and Sandberg's approach to cautionary heuristics would still be defective, because it focuses on adaptation, rather than upon the risk that IGM will disrupt benign causal interdependencies and in doing so produce bad unintended consequences.

Bostrom and Sandberg advocate a heuristic for intervention, which they call the "evolutionary optimality challenge" (EOC).[18] The EOC places the burden of proof on IGM proponents to meet the following adaptationist test: "If the proposed intervention would result in an enhancement, why have we not already evolved to be that way?" The authors propose this optimality criterion because they feel that it reflects the grain of truth in the Master Engineer analogy. The EOC can be based on either or both of the following claims: (1) if X is an adaptation, then X will tend to be optimal from an evolutionary and/or moral standpoint; (2) if X is an adaptation, then manipulating its genetic underpinnings will tend to produce negative phenotypic consequences. Bostrom and Sandberg proceed on the assumption that natural selection is the only important cause of biological traits, which, because they are adaptive, also tend to be functionally and morally optimal. As we have seen, neither is the case, and thus (1) is clearly false and (2) makes no claims about optimality (the EOC moniker notwithstanding). It is simply the reasonable assertion that caution is needed in modifying parts of the genome that code for adaptive elements of the phenotype. The nonlinear interactions between genes and gene networks certainly counsel against the willy-nilly manipulation of sequences coding for highly integrated functions. There is therefore nothing wrong with urging caution about IGM in the context of adaptive traits; the problem with Bostrom and Sandberg's heuristic, however, is that it is focuses perilously on the *wrong set of facts*. As a result, it can lead IGM seriously astray by suggesting *looser* standards for the modification of maladaptive or non-adaptive portions of the genome.

There is no question that even small genetic perturbations, especially early in ontogeny, can wreak havoc on biological function; but this is true *whether or not the target of intervention is an adaptation*. So we should equally caution against the cavalier alteration of *non-adaptive* or *neutral* segments of the genome, which due to "epistasis" (the interaction between genetic loci in relation to their effect on the phenotype) can have comparable or even more serious genetic consequences. What matters for the purposes of assessing the potential negative consequences of IGM is not whether the target of intervention is the underlying cause of an adaptation, but how the target genes are causally connected with other genes and gene products in the unfolding of the organism from embryo to maturity. In other words, our best guess as to the probable effects of IGM should always rest on an assessment of *current causal capacities*—not events in the distant past. Strong adaptationism, which adheres to a backward-looking, purely etiological conception of function, not a current causal conception, sheds little light on this question. To see why this is so, consider that there are two conceptual approaches to function in contemporary biology. The most popular is the "etiological" or "selected effects" version of biological function, which defines a trait's function in relation to its particular selective history.[19] The "causal role" account of function, on the other hand, is concerned not with the genealogy of a trait, but rather its current causal properties.[20] Now for the crucial point: in the context of IGM, the current causal properties of the target "screen off" (i.e., render statistically irrelevant) adaptive etiology with respect to the probability of the unintended negative consequences of intervention. This is not to say that adaptive etiology cannot provide some basic clues about the risks associated with intervention; but a sufficient understanding of current causal capacities (or the co-variance structure between genes and phenotypic traits) renders information about genealogy moot. If I wanted to figure out what my college roommate was up to nowadays, I would give him a call or ask his neighbors; I would most certainly not dig up our college correspondence in an effort to reconstruct the past, merely to make an educated guess at what he might be doing in the present. And yet this is precisely what the EOC would have us do.

At this point, Bostrom and Sandberg might argue that given the limitations of our current knowledge regarding both the general nature and fine-grained details of complex gene networks, we should focus instead on selected effects which are easier to determine than current causal capacities. Were this in fact true, it would at least provide some basis for their adaptationist heuristics. But it is simply not the case that selected effects functions are easier to ascertain than causal role functions; in fact the reverse is probably true.[21] "Just-so stories" of the natural history of a trait may be easier to *concoct* than hypotheses regarding proximate causal dynamics, but this does not make them any more likely to be *accurate*, or to succeed in helping us avoid the negative consequences of intervention. In contrast, mathematical simulations have been used to model nonlinear developmental networks, allowing for specific predictions regarding the effects of mutation, genetic modification, and perturbations in non-genetic factors on the ontogeny of complex traits.[22]

In sum, the EOC is problematic in that it relies on indirect and potentially misleading information about the likely consequences of genetic intervention, while overlooking the developmental harm that could flow from modifying both maladaptive and non-adaptive regions of the genome. One final point: while it is true that the vast majority of "natural" mutations are either maladaptive or neutral,[23] the very point of IGM is that it does *not* mimic the mutational processes of UGM. Its purpose, rather, is to produce targeted, non-random variation in the service of some identifiable goal. Thus, the fact that unassisted genetic variation (i.e., mutation) is only rarely beneficial actually *supports* rather than detracts from the value of IGM.

Bostrom and Sandberg are right to explore the idea of contentful, cautionary heuristics that steer a course between a blanket prohibition on IGM and the vagueness of an admonition to "go slow." They are also correct in their assumption that the needed heuristics must be informed by evolutionary biology. Where they go wrong is in assuming that the key question to ask is whether a trait targeted for IGM is an adaptation. Not all traits are adaptive, not all modifications of adaptations will have negative consequences, and not all modifications of non-adaptive traits will be benign in their effects. In each case, what matters is not adaptive etiology, but the causal relationship between the target trait/gene and other ontogenetic factors, including those features of the organism that we value and wish to preserve.

Cautionary heuristics grounded in causal ontogenetic relationships

My purpose in this chapter is not to develop a thoroughgoing account of the implications of a sound understanding of contemporary evolutionary theory for IGM in humans. Instead, the goal has been to expose some of the misconceptions about evolution that have distorted the debate over genetic modification in general and genetic modification for enhancement in particular. Nevertheless, before concluding I wish to offer an admittedly incomplete list of cautionary heuristics, focusing not on adaptation, but on causal ontogenetic (i.e., developmental) relationships. These rules of thumb are not offered as necessary or sufficient conditions for the permissibility of UGM. Instead, they are an attempt to translate the correct but unhelpfully vague admonition to "go slow" into something more capable of providing concrete guidance for determining whether to pursue a proposed genetic modification for the sake of increasing human well-being. They are intended only to help reduce the risk of what might be called "biological damage." They do not address the possibility that IGM might produce unintended bad social or moral consequences. They are not offered as anything approaching a comprehensive guide to decision-making in the context of IGM. Nevertheless, when taken together, they reflect a proper concern for the risk of unintended biological consequences arising from the genetic modification of complex organisms, while avoiding the misconceptions that the Master engineer analogy encourages. The more of these seven conditions a proposed intervention satisfies and the more fully it satisfies them, the more confident we can be that the risk of unintended bad (biological) consequences has been taken seriously. How serious the failure to satisfy one or more of the seven conditions is will depend upon a number of factors, including, of course, how valuable the intended effects of the genetic modification are and how likely it is that the intervention will produce them.

1. The intervention targets genes at shallower ontogenetic depths, ones that lie "downstream" in the development of the organism from embryo to maturity. Such interventions are less likely to have cascading negative consequences for phenotype.

2. The intervention, if successful, would not produce an enhancement that exceeds the upper bound of the current normal distribution of the trait in question. The idea here is that if there are existing, well-functioning individuals who already possess the trait whose frequency one is trying to increase, then this provides some assurance that the modification will not disrupt benign causal interdependencies. Thus, for example, IGM to increase some aspect of cognitive function for those at the lower end of the current normal range would be preferable to interventions aimed at raising the upper bound of the normal (other things being equal).

3. The intervention's effects are containable to a particular organism. In other words, if there turn out to be bad unintended consequences, the damage will be limited to the individual(s) in which the intervention occurs.

4. The intervention is containable *within* the organism—that is, it involves modifications in a highly modularized system or subsystem

of the organism. Such a modification is less likely to produce unintended spillover effects into other systems or subsystems.

5. The intervention's effects are reversible. If this condition is satisfied, then it will be possible to avoid ongoing damage.

6. The intervention does not entail major morphological changes. The intuition here is that major morphological modifications are more likely to have bad unintended consequences on phenotypic development than minor ones.

7. If the goal of the intervention is to eliminate an undesirable trait, then the *causal role* functions of the trait and its underling genetic substrate should be well understood. This heuristic reflects the recognition that even "bad" traits may have some benign consequences, and that the price of eliminating a bad trait may be prohibitive, depending on its causal connections to other genes and how they in turn affect the phenotype.

Each of these heuristics is designed to reduce the risk of unintended bad consequences in the right way: that is, by focusing on causal relationships in development, rather than on the adaptive etiology of the trait targeted for intervention.

The Precautionary Principle

The pluralistic risk-reduction strategy I have just argued rejects the idea that there is one master principle of risk reduction. It opts instead for a set of cautionary heuristics that reflect various distinct sources of risk in the use of IGM. This approach contrasts sharply with reliance on the Precautionary Principle. Some have invoked the Precautionary Principle in support of a total ban on genetic modification of foods; others have appealed to it as the basis for a ban on all enhancement IGM in humans. In this section I explain how problematic the Precautionary Principle is and argue that the pluralistic approach developed in the preceding section is a better way of addressing the risks of IGM.

The vagueness of the Precautionary Principle

If by "the Precautionary Principle" one means a single cautionary heuristic, there is no such thing. Instead there is at most a vague and capacious schema involving several placeholders that can be filled in to yield a plurality of quite different principles and tremendous controversy as to how they should be filled in. There are two classic statements of the principle in the domain of public international environmental documents. The Rio Declaration on Environment and Regulation (1992) states "the principle" as follows:

In order to protect the environment, the precautionary approach shall be widely applied by States according to their capabilities. Where there are threats of serious or irreversible damage, lack of scientific certainty shall not be used as a reason for postponing cost-effective measures to prevent environmental degradation.[24]

Participants in the 1998 Wingspread conference on the environment issued a statement saying that

When an activity raises threats of harm to human health or the environment precautionary measures should be taken even if some cause and effect relationships are not fully established scientifically.... In this context the proponent of an activity, rather than the public, should bear the burden of proof.[25]

Both formulations are so vague that it is hard to assess them. Nevertheless, the Rio formulation appears considerably weaker than the Wingspread formulation. Taken literally, it only says that the fact it is not possible to predict a harm with "scientific certainty" is not a reason to postpone measures to prevent the harm. It does *not* require prohibition of risky activities; nor does it require fully successful measures to prevent the harms they may cause. Depending on how high the standard of "scientific certainty" is set and what counts as a "serious" risk, one gets quite different results.

The Wingspread statement seems much stronger: it suggests that before a potentially harmful activity is undertaken, those who propose it must *prove* that it is not harmful—that it poses no risk at all. If that is what it means, it is clearly far too constraining as a general principle regarding risk. It would bar us from undertaking even the most beneficial actions if they carried any risk at all. Interpreted more charitably, it would not to apply to risks generally, but only to very serious or perhaps catastrophic risks. Even when understood in this more restrictive fashion, however, the Wingspread principle is problematic, because it focuses only on potential harms, not on benefits. It fails to consider the possibility that in some circumstances—perhaps global warming is an example—*not intervening* carries extreme, perhaps catastrophic risks.

If there is a basic idea that is common to the Rio statement, the Wingspread statement, and many other proposals for a "precautionary approach" to environmental policy, it is something like this: there is to be a very strong presumption in favor of prevention of *harms that could result from human activities*. This explains why some anti-enhancement writers have endorsed the extension of "the precautionary approach" from its home turf in the environmental arena to the case of biomedical enhancements of human beings.

Here we encounter a paradox, however. Further human actions may be indispensable for ameliorating the harms that previous human actions have caused. Once again, global warming provides a plausible example. If we take seriously the idea that there is a strong presumption in favor of preventing harms that result from human activities, then it the principle implies that we must simply acquiesce in the harms that our activities have already produced and refrain from any new actions to mitigate them. Both the harm that we are trying to prevent (the ill effects of global warming) and the harm that our harm prevention efforts may cause (the unintended bad consequences of our response to global warming) are harms caused by human actions.

The maximin interpretation of the Precautionary Principle

In an exceptionally valuable article, Stephen Gardiner has suggested that there is one interpretation of "the precautionary principle" that makes it more plausible.[26] On this interpretation, the precautionary principle is the maximin principle, applied to environmental regulation issues or, in our case, choices about IGM. The maximin principle is a rule for decision-making: one is to choose that option with the best worst outcome.

The consensus among decision-theorists is that the maximin rule is applicable only to decisions under uncertainty, not decisions under risk. Decisions under risk are cases in which one can make reasonable estimates of the probabilities of the outcomes under the various options; decisions under uncertainty are situations in which one cannot make reasonable estimates of the probabilities. The maximin rule applies only in conditions of profound ignorance of the causal relationships relevant to the problem of unintended bad consequences.

It is important to understand that the maximin rule is not the only decision rule for decision-making under uncertainty. It is only plausible to use the maximin rule in those cases of decision-making under uncertainty in which one attaches no value or very little value to benefits above those one would get in the best worst-case scenario. To put the same point differently: to follow the maximin rule is to act as if one were extremely harm averse—as if all that mattered was avoiding harm.

It should be obvious why the maximin interpretation of the precautionary principle is not a plausible candidate for a cautionary heuristic regarding IGM. Neither of the conditions for its applicability apply. First, we do care about gains, not just losses. As I argued in Chapter Two, some enhancements through IGM may be extremely valuable, for all of us. This becomes very clear once we recognize that enhancements may be needed not just to improve our situation relative to the status quo, but also to sustain the goods we now enjoy, but it also applies to cases where an enhancement would lift us far above our present condition. Second, so far as biomedical enhancements in general are concerned, including enhancements through IGM, we are not typically in a situation of decision-making under uncertainty. We already have considerable knowledge of the causal connections that are relevant to assessments of proposed interventions—sufficient knowledge to make reasonable probability estimates in some cases.

Consider, for example, our extensive and growing knowledge of the effects of particular genetic modifications in laboratory animals with whom we share the genes in question, as well as our knowledge of the phenotypic effects of genetic mutations in humans. For particular proposed genetic modifications, this knowledge will sometimes suffice for making reasonable estimates of the probabilities of the outcome. Relying on a principle that only makes sense if our ignorance is total makes no sense in a situation in which we have considerable knowledge regarding some particular interventions. Our decisions should be based on an appreciation of the extent of our knowledge.

The maximin interpretation of the Precautionary Principle, like the bright line prohibition strategy, not only overestimates the current state of our ignorance but also ignores the fact that our knowledge is growing. The bright line prohibition strategy and the maximin rule have something else in common: they are both not only knowledge-insensitive but also *knowledge-thwarting*: they pose serious obstacles to gaining knowledge that is clearly relevant to the issue of risk. Following the bright line prohibition guarantees that our knowledge of the probable effects of enhancements will remain limited, because it forbids us to undertake even the least risky enhancements. If we follow the maximin interpretation of the Precautionary Principle, we are forbidden to undertake any experimental intervention whose worst possible outcome is worse than the worst possible outcome of not intervening, even if neither outcome is very bad. In both cases, the risk-reducing strategy bars us from obtaining knowledge that is relevant to our assessments of risk.

I do not pretend to have plumbed the depths of the complex debate over the Precautionary Principle. Nevertheless, I think it is fair to say that so far no one has succeeded in formulating a version of the precautionary principle that is both plausible and sufficiently determinate to guide policy. My surmise is that further efforts to try to formulate a better precautionary principle is not a good investment of energy, because it is highly improbable that any single risk-reduction principle can do the job. It is more likely that a plurality of cautionary heuristics will be needed. One key desideratum is that they should be knowledge-sensitive: they should help us to take into account both the limitations and the extent of our knowledge as we grapple with the risk of unintended bad consequences. Another is that they should be knowledge-encouraging, or at least not knowledge-inhibiting.

Conclusion

The most serious worry about biomedical enhancement is the risk of bad unintended consequences. How we frame the issue of risk matters, as does our choice of strategies for reducing risk. The use of faulty analogies such as that of a Master Engineer or a Seamless Web is an obstacle to framing the issue judiciously. It is also an impediment to identifying sound risk-reduction strategies. If one ignores the facts of evolutionary biology and proceeds dogmatically on the assumption of ubiquitous extreme connectedness, one may be drawn toward the Precautionary Principle. But once we see that there is no good reason to accept the extreme connectedness assumption and considerable evidence against it, the proposal to proceed as if all we cared about was ensuring against the worst outcome and as if we had no knowledge of the probabilities of the outcomes of our action looks implausible. As our knowledge of the causal relationships involved in the development of the human organism increases, we will be able to undertake enhancements, including ones that utilize the genetic modification of embryos or gametes, that do not involve excessive risk, so long as we adhere to cautionary heuristics that reflect both what we know about evolution and a healthy awareness that our knowledge is limited.

Perhaps the greatest flaw of the analogy of evolution as a Master Engineer is that it ignores the fact that organisms not only react to their environments but also shape them. As biologists have long recognized, adaptations are not to ecological niches as keys are to locks.[27] Rather, organisms engage in a reciprocal and co-defining relationship with their selective environment.[28] As organisms go, humans are niche-constructors par excellence. They have been transforming the face of the planet for thousands of years, although the technological revolutions of the twentieth century have marked the anthropogenic alteration of global ecosystems at a scale, rate, and intensity that dwarfs the entire history of human impact combined.[29] Given the furious pace of recent cultural niche construction, it is not surprising that our biology has had little chance to catch up. IGM could help us adjust to the new design problems that we are rapidly creating for ourselves.[30]

Given the severe biological and moral constraints of "unassisted" evolution, and given that intentional genetic modification has the potential to avoid these limitations, we have good reason to develop the capacity for IGM. But evolutionary theory also helps us appreciate the functional intricacies of complex organisms, and hence the seriousness of the risk that IGM, undertaken without sufficient knowledge of causal relationships, could result in the unwitting disruption of important ontogenetic processes. The right place to begin making decisions about using or refraining from IGM is a proper appreciation of the limits of UGM and a frank acknowledgement of the current limits of our knowledge regarding the causal structure of molecular development—not with a distorted picture of evolution that stacks the deck against IGM.

In this chapter I have exposed and dismantled some key misframings of the problem of unintended bad consequences. I have also offered a set of cautionary heuristics to guide difficult decisions about what many regard as the most risky mode of biomedical enhancement, the deliberate modification of human genes in embryos or gametes. Cautionary heuristics of the sort considered here are not algorithms for making enhancement decisions. They do not eliminate the need for judgment. Nor are they intended as timeless guidelines for decision-making. Julian Savulescu has noted that, generally speaking, the value of heuristics consists in their being proxies for more accurate knowledge about the matter at hand. If this is so, Savulescu concludes, then as our knowledge of human biology increases, the need for reliance on these heuristics may diminish.

The value of heuristics does not depend solely on our ignorance of the scientific facts, however. It also depends on our fallibility. Relying on them can help to counter tendencies to overestimate our knowledge or to unduly discount the risks that our decisions may entail. If, as seems likely, there will be potent commercial pressures to develop biomedical enhancement technologies, there will be a tendency on the part of some actors to overestimate benefits and underestimate risks. In addition, scientific experts, like other experts, are subject to incentives that can push them toward overestimating the extent of their knowledge. Adherence to a set of cautionary heuristics of the sort sketched in this chapter could do something to mitigate the risks to which our risk-coping behavior is subject.

Sound cautionary heuristics only mitigate risk if they are actually followed, however. The next step in developing an effective response to the risks that biomedical enhancement poses, therefore, would be to begin the hard task of thinking about how to ensure that key players in the process of developing biomedical enhancements take the heuristics seriously. That would require institutionalizing the heuristics— developing a consensus on them and then building them into the practices of the biomedical research community. It is beyond the scope of this book to take even the first tentative steps in this direction. My aim has been more modest: to articulate a set of cautionary heuristics that can provide a focus for discussions that will eventually engage the issue of institutionalizing a responsible strategy for reducing the risks of the enhancement enterprise. In the final chapter, I do more to illustrate the importance of thinking institutionally about the challenges of biomedical enhancement. There I identify one central aspect of the problem of justice in enhancement and offer a detailed institutional proposal for coping with it. Before concluding the book with that concrete, practical

206 Unintended Bad Consequences

discussion, however, the next chapter grapples with what some consider the most disturbing prospect of biomedical enhancement: the possibility that it may lead to a fundamental disruption in our moral framework, by exploding our most basic assumptions about moral status—about which kinds of beings count the most, morally speaking.

Notes

1. Michael Sandel (2007), *The Case Against Perfection: Ethics in the Age of Genetic Engineering* (Cambridge, MA: Harvard University Press), p. 96; President's Council on Bioethics (2002), *Human Cloning and Human Dignity: An Ethical Inquiry* (Washington, DC: National Bioethics Advisory Commission), p. ix.
2. Sandel 2007, supra note 1, (italics added).
3. This section draws on Russell Powell and Allen Buchanan (forthcoming), "Breaking Evolution's Chains: The Promise of Enhancement By Design," in *Enhancing Human Capacities*, Ruud ter Muelen, Julian Savulescu, and Guy Kahane (eds.) (Oxford: Oxford University Press).
4. Here and throughout, by "genetic modification" I mean germline changes, that is, modifications of genes in embryos or gametes (sperm or eggs), changes that are expected to be passed on to the next generation, rather than somatic cell genetic modifications, as occurs, for example, when genes are inserted into bone marrow for therapeutic purposes.
5. President's Council on Bioethics (2002), *Beyond Therapy* (Washington, DC: National Bioethics Advisory Commission).
6. The nature and use of teleological language in biology has been the subject of controversy since Darwin's time. While T.H. Huxley proclaimed that "teleology...had received its deathblow at Mr. Darwin's hands," Asa Gray lauded "Darwin's great service to natural science in bringing it back to teleology." Quoted in M. Ruse (2003), *Darwin and Design: Does Evolution Have a Purpose?* (Cambridge, MA: Cambridge University Press), p. 91.
   Regardless of where one stands in this methodological debate, there is little question that Darwinian theory obliterated any hopes that final causation would play an irreducible metaphysical role in the evolutionary process.
7. N. Bostrom and A. Sandberg (2009), "The Wisdom of Nature: An Evolutionary Heuristic for Human Enhancement," in *Human Enhancement*, Julian Savulescu and Nick Bostrom (eds.) (Oxford University Press).
8. It is an "axiom" of cancer research that tumor formation is driven by both oncogenes (dominant growth-enhancing genes) and mutations in growth-inhibitory genes, hundreds of which have thus far been discovered. See I. B. Weinstein (2002), "Addiction to Oncogenes—the Achilles Heal of Cancer," *Science* 297: 63–64.

9. See E. Todd Schroeder *et al.* (2007), "Hormonal regulators of muscle and metabolism in aging (HORMA): design and conduct of a complex, double masked multicenter trial," *Clinical Trials* 4(5): 560–571.
10. R.N. Brandon (2006), "The principle of drift: Biology's first law," *Journal of Philosophy* CIII(7): 319–335.
11. See R.N. Brandon and M.D. Rausher (1996), "Testing Adaptationism: A Comment on Orzack and Sober," *The American Naturalist* 148(1): 189–201.
12. For an overview of this debate, see S.H. Orzack and E. Sober (1994), "How (Not) to Test an Optimality Model," *Trends in Ecology and Evolution* 9: 265–267, and the reply by Brandon and Rausher 1996, supra note 11.
13. See Roger Sansom (2003), "Constraining the Adaptationism Debate," *Biology and Philosophy* 18: 493–512.
14. On the potential of genetic enhancement to expand the range of the humanly possible, see A. Buchanan (2009), "Enhancement and Human Nature," *Bioethics* 23(3): 141–150.
15. See Joan Silk and Robert Boyd (2006), *How Humans Evolved* (W.W. Norton and Co.).
16. See e.g. A.P. Galvani and M. Slatkin (2003), "Evaluating plague and smallpox as historical selective pressures for the CCR5-Delta 32 HIV resistance allele," *Proceedings of the National Academy of Sciences USA* 100: 15276–15279.
17. See R. Amundson (1994), "Two Concepts of Constraint: Adaptationism and the Challenge from Developmental Biology," *Philosophy of Science* 61: 556–578. For a critique of strong adaptationism, see J. Beatty (1984), "Pluralism and Panselectionism," in P.D. Asquith and P. Kitcher (eds.), *Philosophy of Science Association* (East Lansing, MI).
18. See Bostrom and Sandberg (2009), supra note 7.
19. See, for example, K. Neander (1991), "Functions as Selected Effects: The Conceptual Analyst's Defense," *Philosophy of Science* 58: 168–184.
20. See R. Amundson G. Lauder (1994), "Function without purpose: The uses of causal role function in evolutionary biology," *Biology and Philosophy* 9: 443–469.
21. See ibid.
22. See, for example, H.F. Nijhout (2003), "The control of growth," *Development* 130: 5863–5867.
23. J.C. Fay, G.J. Wyckoff and C.I. Wu (2001), "Positive and negative selection on the human genome," *Genetics* 158: 1227–1234.
24. Rio Declaration on Environment and Development, UN Doc. A/CONF.151/26 (vol. I); 31 ILM 874 (1992).
25. Wingspread Statement on the Precautionary Principle (1998), http://www.gdrc.org/u-gov/precaution-3.html.
26. S.M. Gardiner (2006), "A Core Precautionary Principle," *Journal of Political Philosophy* 14(1): 33–60.

208 Unintended Bad Consequences

27. This was first pointed out in a classic paper by R.C. Lewontin (1982), "Organism & Environment: Learning, Development, Culture," Henry Plotkin (ed.), New York: John Wiley, pp. 151–170.
28. J.J. Odling-Smee, K.N. Laland, and M.W. Feldman (2003), *Niche Construction: The Neglected Process in Evolution* (New Jersey: Princeton University Press).
29. J. McNeil (2001), Something New under the Sun: An Environmental History of the Twentieth-Century World (W.W. Norton & Co.).
30. Even if it were the case that IGM technology would reduce our long-term prospects of survival (when in fact the opposite appears to be true), it would still not follow that we should refrain from developing it. For individuals and for humanity collectively, some risk of death may be worth taking, if the gains are great enough. Everyone who drives a car, or flies in a plane, or for that matter, takes a shower, recognizes this at the level of individual survival. Human well-being simply does not reduce to maximizing the chances of survival either at the individual or the species level.

CHAPTER SEVEN

Moral Status and Enhancement

Moral Status, Moral Equality, and the Prospect of Enhancement

From the standpoint of justice, the most common worry about enhancement is this: if enhancements are expensive and therefore available only to the better off, existing *distributive* inequalities—inequalities in resources, opportunities, or welfare—will worsen. The economically advantaged will become biologically advantaged to boot. In Chapter Eight, I consider an institutional innovation that could ameliorate the problem of injustice in access to enhancements. In the present chapter, I focus on a more profound worry about inequality: the emergence of a group of beings (the enhanced) who would have a *higher* moral status than that possessed by normal human beings now.

The thought that enhancement might produce a morally bifurcated world of (mere) *persons* and *postpersons*[1] is deeply disquieting. It would be threatening from the perspective of the unenhanced (the mere persons), who would no longer enjoy the highest moral status, as they did when there were only persons and nonpersons ("lower animals"). The prospect of a distinction between (mere) persons and (higher moral status) postpersons is disturbing for another reason: it challenges the very widely held *Moral Equality Assumption*—the assumption that all who have the characteristics that are sufficient for being a person have the same moral status.[2]

The terms "moral status" and "moral standing" are sometimes used interchangeably, but in the analysis that follows I will distinguish them. I will say that a being has moral standing if it counts morally, in its own right. For Bentham, sentient beings count morally in their own right.

For Kant, only persons, beings with the capacity for practical rationality, have moral standing. On both views, moral standing is not a comparative notion. Moral status, in contrast, is a comparative notion. Two beings can both have moral standing, but one may be of a higher moral status.

The idea that different beings with moral standing have different moral statuses is common to otherwise divergent moral theories. It is implicit in much pre-theoretical, commonsense moral thinking as well. A being's moral status can make a difference as to whether its behavior is subject to moral evaluation, how it ought to be treated, whether it has rights, and perhaps what kinds of rights it has. In moral views that include a plurality of moral statuses, it is human beings, or at least human beings who are persons, that are thought to occupy the highest status.

On some accounts, the concept of human rights is an important articulation of the idea of equal moral status.[3] Some participants in the enhancement debate have gone so far as to say that enhancements might render the concept of human rights obsolete.[4] They worry about the obsolescence of the concept of human rights because they believe that enhancements could result in beings that were not human beings, and apparently assume that the concept of human rights applies only to human beings. Those who have expressed this worry have tended to use "human rights" and "the rights of persons" interchangeably. They have failed to acknowledge that some human beings (i.e., members of the species, Homo sapiens), including the profoundly demented and infants, do not have some of the characteristics that moral philosophers typically attribute to persons and that are thought to ground the distinctive rights that persons have. Nor have they considered the possibility that at least some of the rights that are called human rights are more properly described as "persons' rights." Nevertheless, their basic concern can be reframed to take the relevant distinctions into account: will enhancements lead to the obsolescence of persons and hence of the concept of the distinctive rights that persons have?

To grasp this second concern, we need to distinguish between two scenarios. In the first, persons are eventually completely replaced, through the sustained use of biomedical enhancement technologies, by a higher sort of being, postpersons. No mere persons remain; the concept of human rights, understood as rights distinctive of (mere) persons, becomes a concept without application.

Presumably, the new, enhanced beings will have rights appropriate to their capacities; call them *postpersons' rights*. If that is so, then there appears to be no problem. One concept of rights loses application and another comes into play. Postpersons will have no cause to regret the obsolescence of the concept of human rights.[5]

In the second scenario, some human beings are enhanced to the point of becoming "postpersons," but others are not. Under these conditions, there seems to be a genuine worry. Even if the concept of human rights (understood as the distinctive rights of persons) still applies to the unenhanced, it will be incapable of playing the distinctive moral role we assign to it now: it will no longer convey the idea that all who satisfy the conditions that are sufficient for personhood have the same moral status. In a world in which there are beings who have all the capacities that confer human rights, but also higher capacities conferring a distinctive set of rights, the assertion that all persons have human rights will not have the moral force it does now. Even if mere persons retain their human rights, the *significance* of their having them will have diminished, because the Moral Equality Assumption will not obtain.

This chapter explores the implications of enhancement for moral status and for the concept of human rights. I will argue for six conclusions. (1) In a world in which some are enhanced and some or not, the concept of human rights, far from being obsolete, would be even more important than it is now. (2) The idea of a moral status higher than that of persons is dubious, given a plausible understanding of the concept of moral status; so the prospect of enhancement does not present a serious threat to the Moral Equality Assumption. (3) Even if we grant the dubious assumption that the emergence of beings with a moral status higher than that of persons is possible, their existence would not extinguish whatever rights the unenhanced have by virtue of being persons. (4) Given the history and persistence of racism, there is a serious risk that the enhanced would treat the unenhanced as if they had a lower moral status, even *if* they do not. (5) Even if enhancements did not create beings with a higher moral status, or foster a mistaken perception of unequal moral statuses, they might result in a conflict of legitimate interests between the enhanced and the unenhanced, and a just accommodation of these conflicting interests might involve restrictions of *some* of the rights of the unenhanced. (6) The possibility that enhancements could mandate such a two-tiered system of rights is a serious moral cost that ought to be taken into account in our decisions regarding the pursuit of enhancement technologies. Exploring the implications of enhancement for moral status can illuminate the choices we may have to make about biomedical enhancements, but it can also spur us to develop a clearer understanding of what moral status is and of the relationship between moral status, rights, personhood, and human nature.

Enhancement, Human Nature, and Human Rights

Some bioethicists, including Leon Kass, Erik Parens, and Francis Fukayama, express the worry about enhancement producing beings with a higher moral status in terms of human nature: they see enhancements as creating beings who are not human beings, but who are superior to humans in ways that are or might be thought to be sufficient for having a higher moral status. Others, including Jeff McMahan, think the possibility of the emergence of beings with a higher moral status and its moral implications can be framed without recourse to the concept of human nature.[6]

Although Kass, Parens, and Fukayama think it is obvious that enhancement could create posthumans (beings whose nature was not human),[7] others, including Norman Daniels, are skeptical.[8] To determine which view is correct, we need a workable but non-question-begging definition of human nature. For purposes of the present discussion, I will rely on the definition I offered in Chapter Four.

Human nature is a set of characteristics (1) that most beings that are uncontroversially human have at this point in biological and cultural evolution (and have had throughout what is uncontroversially thought to be human [as opposed to prehuman] history); (2) that are relatively recalcitrant to being expunged or significantly altered by education, training, and indoctrination; and (3) that play a significant role in explanations of widespread human behavior and in explanations of differences between humans and other animals.

I argued in Chapter Four that on this definition of human nature, the cumulative effect of a series of enhancements, undertaken on a large scale, could be the emergence of *posthumans*—beings sufficiently different from us that it would make sense to regard them as other than human beings, as having a nature different from that of human nature. As difficult as it may be for us to imagine what sort of changes would require the recognition of a new species, we cannot dismiss the possibility. My aim here is not to argue conclusively for the claim that biomedical enhancements might eventually result in posthumans. Instead, I only hope to have made this possibility plausible enough to motivate the two questions with which I am concerned. (1) If enhancement did result in posthumans, what implications would this have for the concept of human rights: would it make that concept obsolete, as some have claimed; and, if it did, would this be a moral catastrophe, as they have intimated? (2) Could the emergence of posthumans result in there being a moral status higher than that of persons and hence require a rejection of the widely held Moral Equality Assumption, according to which all who have the characteristics sufficient for being persons are of equal moral status? In the remainder of this section, I will answer the first question; in the next section, I will answer the second. In the third section "The idea of a higher, 'postperson' moral status," I will argue that even if enhancements did not produce beings with a higher moral status, it might result in a system of *unequal rights* and that this would be a significant moral cost that should be taken into account in deciding whether to pursue enhancements. Whether a system of unequal rights implies unequal moral status depends on which rights are implicated in moral status and, I shall argue, it is not clear that any existing account of moral status (or of rights) can answer that question.

Those who worry that the emergence of posthumans would render the concept of human rights obsolete assume that human rights are rights we have *by virtue of our humanity*. What these critics of enhancement have failed to notice is that in human rights discourse the claim that there are certain rights we have by virtue of our humanity serves two functions: it conveys the idea that the possession of these rights does not depend upon their being recognized in law (in that sense, they are "natural rights" not "positive rights"); and it signals inclusiveness or universality, by implying that these rights are not limited to any subset of human beings such as males, whites, or people of this or that religion, ethnicity, or race. On this understanding of the claim that human rights are rights we have by virtue of our humanity, and regardless of whether "humanity" refers to humans as members of a biological species or to persons, the claim is merely that humanity is a *sufficient* condition for having these rights, not that it is a necessary condition.[9] Thus it could be true that we human beings have certain rights simply by virtue of our humanity, but it could also be true that there are other beings—for example, nonhuman forms of intelligent life on other planets—who also have them, if those beings also had whatever it takes to confer (what we call) human rights. If "humanity" refers to personhood, rather than to membership in the human biological species, and if we came to know that there were persons who were not of our biological species, then we might decide that what we have called human rights would be more accurately called *persons' rights*. If "humanity" refers to our biological species, it might be that those features of our biology that are sufficient for having what we call human rights are shared by extraterrestrials of another species. The point is that a plausible understanding of the claim that human rights are rights we have by virtue of our humanity does *not* imply that the concept of human rights is applicable only to human beings.[10] But if that is so, then the emergence of posthumans, even if this were accompanied by the extinction of human beings, would *not* entail that the concept of human rights would no longer be applicable. The concept of human rights would still be applicable if posthumans had the capabilities or interests that ground (what we now call) human rights.[11]

Yet surely at least some of the rights we now call human rights are rights only for *human* persons. After all, at least part of what respect for human rights achieves is the protection of the conditions for a decent human life, under the conditions in which humans now generally find themselves. The point is that *the rights we now have as human persons reflect the way we are now*: not just our biological characteristics, but also the interests we have and the threats we now face, given the sorts of institutions we live under. If there are nonhuman persons, then presumably the conditions for a decent life for them are different, and to that extent their rights will differ also. If enhancement changed us sufficiently, then at least some of the rights we now call human rights might not apply to us and other rights might apply. So, in that sense, enhancement could perhaps lead to the obsolescence of human rights—if no (mere) human beings remained.

As I have already suggested, however, that would not be a moral catastrophe. Rather, it would be morally fitting. If we now have certain rights by virtue of our humanity or by virtue of the conditions under which we now live, then when we are posthumans we will have whatever rights are appropriate for posthumans. So, when bioethicists worry about the obsolescence of human rights, they must (or at least should) have something else in mind than the possibility that if we become posthumans we will have posthuman rights. Perhaps they are worried about the situation in which some are enhanced to the point of being other than human and some are not.[12]

The importance of human rights in a world of humans and posthumans

In a world in which some but not all were enhanced to the point of becoming posthumans, the concept of human rights, far from becoming obsolete, would become even more important. The concept of human rights is a threshold concept, not a scalar one. What matters from the standpoint of the ascription of human rights is whether an individual has certain capabilities or interests; the fact that other individuals have them to a greater degree is irrelevant. Similarly, according to theories that accord moral status (or the highest moral status) to persons, understood as beings who have the capacity for practical rationality or for engaging in practices of mutual accountability,[13] what matters is whether one has the capacity in question. Once the threshold is reached, *how well* one reasons practically or *how well* one engages in practices of mutual accountability does not affect one's moral status.

It is precisely because the concept of human rights, like that of moral status, is a threshold concept that human rights would be extremely important in a world in which some but not all were enhanced. In fact, we already live in such a world: the world's worst-off people are un-enhanced in some respects compared with the best off. On average, people in "developed" countries are taller, stronger, healthier, better able to produce and create more, better able to develop their talents, better able to promote their own values, and longer-lived than people in "less-developed" countries. What we call "economic development" consists of a complex set of processes by which human beings come to be enhanced in certain respects; that is, they gain capacities they previously did not possess and some of their existing capacities are augmented.[14] In a world in which gaps in economic development have resulted in some being enhanced (in some respects) while others are not, human rights discourse is of critical importance, for two reasons. First, it conveys the idea that individuals have basic moral entitlements that ground duties on the part of others, regardless of whether those individuals are "enhanced" or not. Second, it is now widely thought to encompass the notion that these basic entitlements include access to the resources (such as education) that are needed for participating effectively in the processes of development—for becoming "enhanced." For these reasons, the concept of human rights would be all the more valuable in a world in which the uses of biotechnology exacerbated the current gap between the enhanced and the unenhanced. Thus the anxious prediction by Fukuyama, Parens, and Annas that enhancement might make the concept of human rights obsolete is not only mistaken, but ironic, because it rests on a failure to appreciate the distinctive functions and value of that concept.

The Idea of a Higher, "PostPerson" Moral Status

I have argued that, although our concept of human nature may be capacious enough to accommodate the kinds of biomedical enhancements that are now most widely discussed, we cannot dismiss the idea that biomedical enhancements might eventually result in posthumans: beings so different from us that the term "human being" no longer applied to them, and that such beings might have rights that are different from human rights. Now I consider a different question: could biomedical enhancements eventually produce post*persons*, beings with a higher status than that of persons? Enhancements that produced posthumans would not necessarily produce postpersons; that this is so is clear from the possibility of nonhuman extraterrestrial persons. If personhood depends upon having a particular set of capacities, not upon having a particular morphology or a particular set of neurological structures or a particular biological lineage, then, as I have already noted, nonhuman persons are a possibility. The prospect of the enhancement of human beings resulting eventually in posthumans is not difficult to understand, but their resulting in post*persons* is another matter. If the idea of beings with basic moral rights, over and above those possessed by persons, makes sense, then a world in which there were persons and postpersons would be a world in which the Moral Equality Assumption would be false, even if the concept of human rights, understood as rights of (mere) persons, still had application and was still of great moral importance.

In contrast to the idea of posthumans, it is not clear whether the notion of postpersons makes sense. Merely augmenting the characteristics that make a being a person doesn't seem to be the sort of thing that could confer higher moral status. If a person's capacity for practical rationality or for engaging in practices of mutual accountability or for conceiving of herself as an agent with interests persisting over time were increased, the result presumably would be an enhanced person, not a new kind of being with a higher moral status than that of person. After all, some human persons are already better than others at practical reasoning, are morally better, or are better able to envision their future existence, but that doesn't mean they have a higher moral status.

The point is that equality of moral status of the sort we associate with personhood can accommodate many inequalities, including inequalities in the very characteristics that confer moral status. That is what it means to say that the concept of moral status is a threshold concept. So it is hard to imagine how enhancement could create beings with a higher moral status than that of person.

Of course, we must take care not to confuse a failure of imagination with conceptual incoherence. Yet how can we explore the moral implications of what we cannot imagine?

Interesting

For now, let us simply bracket the problem of imagining what sorts of new characteristics would confer a higher moral status than that of persons and consider *the moral structure* of a world in which such a higher status existed. Suppose there were three moral statuses.

1. Postpersons, with Rights R1–R6 (postpersons' rights)
2. Human persons (as we are now), with Rights R1–R4 (persons' rights)
3. Nonhuman, nonperson animals, with Rights R1–R2 or with a moral status that confers serious constraints on how they may be treated, though not rights)

For many of us, the moral universe already includes the inequality of moral status marked by the distinction between 2 and 3: we think it is perfectly plausible to say that humans (or at least those humans who are persons) have a distinct, and higher moral status than, say, rats.

Different moral statuses versus variable moral considerability

There are two main philosophical theories (or families of theories) that purport to explain the difference in moral status marked by the distinction between 2 and 3: interest-based accounts, and intrinsic moral worth, or respect-based accounts. According to interest-based accounts, the moral status of a being depends, roughly, upon how much good its life involves.[15] "Good" here refers to the well-being of the individual in question, understood as comprising various interests. This view implies, among other things, that the wrongness of killing a being depends upon how much good will thereby be lost.

It is not clear that the interest-based view can support the morally momentous distinction between persons and nonpersons that is implicated in the commonsense idea that nonhuman animals have a lower moral *status*. Instead, the interest-based view, properly understood, seems to be a kind of debunking of the idea of different moral statuses, properly speaking, and a recommendation to replace it with something more like *a continuum or gradient of moral considerability*. One can imagine a range of interests, but it is harder to imagine a sharp division between types of interests that would justify the moral status difference that is represented by the distinction between 2 and 3. The concept of moral status appears to be a threshold concept and because it is, the idea of greater or lesser good that the interest-based view operates with seems ill suited to it.

According to the respect-based account stemming from Kant's moral philosophy, all beings that possess certain capacities have an intrinsic moral worth that in some sense confers *inviolability*. Here there is no room for the idea of degrees of moral considerability of the sort that the interest-based account apparently must recognize. Contemporary contractualist moral theorists ground intrinsic moral worth in the capacity to engage in mutual accountability through giving and heeding reasons.[16] Proponents of the respect-based view can admit that there may be a fuzzy lower boundary for this threshold: that it may be difficult to judge whether some human beings (for example very young children or cognitively impaired adults) have the capacity for mutual accountability. Nonetheless, the respect-based view can identify uncontroversial cases of individuals possessing the capacity in question. More important, it can explain why any being who clearly has the capacity in question is owed *equal* respect and hence why having the psychological and motivational characteristics that constitute the capacity to a higher degree does not confer higher moral status. On contractualist understandings of the respect-based view, the same capacity that is said to confer moral status also is the source of the moral principles that give content to the recognition of moral status, including those pertaining to the rights that accompany the moral status of person.

On the respect-based view, it makes sense to say that even though the characteristics that constitute the capacity that confers moral status admit of degree, once one has the capacity, having those characteristics to a higher degree is morally irrelevant. In contrast, if having a good is what confers moral considerability, then having a higher good or being capable of greater well-being should always be relevant to how one ought to be treated. The fact that the respect-based view can explain why having the characteristics that confer moral status to a higher degree does not confer higher status seems to me to be a significant difference between the respect-based view and the interest-based view. Accordingly, the respect-based view seems better suited to provide an account of moral status, understood as a threshold concept, than the latter.

It might be argued that there is another, perhaps even more fundamental, difference between the interest-based view and the respect-based view. The respect-based view seems more plausible as an account of the moral status of persons, simply because it, unlike the interest-based view, focuses on persons. The interest-based view focuses not on persons, but on interests as the ultimate objects of moral concern. In that sense, it is committed to the somewhat odd view that persons, as such, have no moral status: that the phrase "persons have a moral status higher than that of animals" is really a misleading way of saying that "certain interests are so morally important that it is appropriate to treat those beings whose interests they are as if they had a higher moral status." So, if it is a requisite of a plausible theory of moral status that it makes straightforward sense of the idea that persons have moral status, it is not clear that the interest-based view is even in the running.[17]

Can we imagine beings with a higher moral status than that of persons?

If we assume the perspective of the interest-based view, it is *not* hard to imagine how biomedical enhancements could eventually produce beings of greater moral considerability: all we have to imagine is beings whose interests were "higher" than ours, in something like the way most of us now believe that our interests are "higher" than those of rats. For example, if the enhanced beings had psychological capacities that allowed them to have richer sources of well-being than we are capable of, then in that sense they would have "higher" interests and would be capable of greater good. But if I am right in concluding that the interest-based view cannot explain differences in moral status, as opposed to differences in moral considerability (because the concept of moral status is a threshold concept), then being able to imagine beings with "higher" interests than ours does *not* show that we can imagine beings with a higher moral status than that of persons.

From the perspective of the respect-based view, beings with a good that is as much "higher" than ours as ours is compared to that of rats does nothing whatsoever to clarify the idea of a higher moral status. Nor does the possibility of beings that are *more skillful* at engaging in practices of mutual accountability. According to the respect-based view on the contractualist interpretation, what matters is whether one has the capacity for mutual accountability, not one's excellence in exercising that capacity. So if the question is whether biomedical enhancements could eventually produce beings with a higher moral status than that of persons, where we take the idea of moral status as a threshold concept seriously, there is a serious obstacle to answering it: we seem unable to imagine the possibility in question. To put the same point somewhat differently, from the perspective of the respect-based view, it is hard to imagine what a *higher threshold*—one that required a higher moral status—would be like. It does not seem plausible to say that it would consist simply of higher levels of the same characteristics that now constitute the threshold the respect-based view employs. In the absence of an account of what the higher threshold would be like, the claim that there could be beings at a higher threshold who would have a higher moral status is not convincing.

Loss of status in the face of a superior alternative?

Perhaps we can think through the implications of adding a third moral status to our world, in spite of the fact that we find it difficult to imagine what sorts of new characteristics might ground the new, higher status represented by 3. *Consider* an analogy. Suppose that rats evolved before humans. It seems clear that whatever moral status rats had on pre-human earth was not diminished by the emergence of humans. It would have been wrong for space travelers who were nonhuman persons to torture rats on pre-human earth for fun, just as it is wrong for us to treat rats that way now. It seems, then, that the mere emergence of beings with superior moral status (if we can make sense of that) would not *by itself* affect the moral status of existing beings. So even if biotechnology eventually yields enhancements that are so radical as to call for a new, higher moral status category for the enhanced, the moral status of the unenhanced would not *thereby* be diminished.

Here it might be objected that there is a sense in which the advent of postpersons *would* diminish the moral status of (mere) persons. If the nonuniversal use of enhancements led to the emergence of beings who are radically superior to us in moral virtue and intelligence, and who had interests that were as much more complex than ours as our interests are compared to the interests of rats, then it would be permissible for them to sacrifice us for their sake, in cases where tragic choices must be made. If, as many presumably now believe, many rats may be killed to save the life of one person, then surely two or perhaps more mere persons could be permissibly killed to save one postperson. In that sense, the moral status of persons would be diminished if enhancements produced postpersons.[18] (For those whose intuitions are stimulated by the ethics of rail transport: consider a trolley problem with mere persons on one track and postpersons on the other.)

Inviolability and the moral status of persons

This objection can be met, if (1) being a person confers the moral status of *inviolability* and if (2) inviolability, properly understood, is a threshold concept. On this view, meeting the requirements for being a person confers inviolability and that is what counts; having the characteristics that confer personhood to a higher degree does not confer greater inviolability. So, whatever exceptions there are to the assertion that persons may not be sacrificed for the sake of other persons applies *equally* to all who qualify as persons, mere persons and postpersons included. The respect-based view includes the idea that all who have the relevant capacity have equal moral worth and that beings of equal moral worth are equally inviolable.[19]

A more sophisticated objection would run as follows. Even those who claim that persons are inviolable acknowledge, albeit reluctantly, that inviolability has its limit in "supreme emergency" cases: that even the most fundamental rights of a person can be permissibly infringed in order to avert a moral catastrophe, such as the violent deaths of a great many innocent people. If the inviolability of persons is not absolute, however, then surely there can be circumstances in which it would be permissible to sacrifice mere persons for the sake of postpersons, in tragic choice situations.[20]

Perhaps a plausible understanding of the inviolability of persons would allow for the possibility that even the most basic rights of persons, including even the right to life, can be infringed in a supreme emergency, a tragic choice situation where the deaths of a great many innocent persons can be avoided only by killing a few innocent persons. But from the fact that inviolability is limited *in this way* it does not follow that the lives of mere persons count for less than those of postpersons. One can consistently acknowledge that there are extreme cases in which inviolability can be overridden, while denying that differences in the nature of the interests or capacities of the beings involved justify the exception. On this threshold understanding of inviolability, the justification for sacrificing some persons for the sake of others is not that the latter have higher interests or capacities, but some other principle, such as that when the most basic rights are at stake, massive violations of persons' rights ought to be avoided, even if this means violating the rights of a few. If this is the right way to understand the inviolability of persons, then the emergence of postpersons would not diminish the moral status of persons. The lives of all who meet the requirements for personhood and the rights it confers, mere persons as well as postpersons, would count equally when tragic choices must be made.

This understanding of inviolability explains the intuition that if an innocent *person* may be sacrificed to save the lives of a great many *persons*, the choice should *not* be made on the basis of any judgment that the person who is to be sacrificed is inferior in some way to those who will be saved. Justifying the decision to sacrifice the one for the many in that way would fail to show the equal respect to which all persons are entitled; it would be a denial of their equal status as persons.

It would be better, on this view, to use a fair lottery to choose the one to be sacrificed, than to rank persons according to some standard of worth or excellence and then sacrifice the person who scored lowest. Similarly, in the bifurcated world we are attempting to imagine, if all persons are inviolable simply by virtue of their being persons, then, if tragic choices must be made, the lives of postpersons should *not* count for more than those of persons. Even if it were true that the death of postpersons involves greater loss of the good because of the "higher" nature of their interests or capacities, it would still not follow that their lives count more. The threshold view of inviolability excludes taking such considerations into account.

My aim here is not to try to provide a theory of supreme emergency exceptions to the inviolability of persons. I have entertained the idea that there are such exceptions, because the more sophisticated of the two objections considered above argues that if such exceptions exist, then those who affirm the inviolability of persons are thereby committed to acknowledging that the lives of postpersons would count for more than those of persons. That inference, I have argued, is invalid, if the inviolability of persons is a threshold concept. Moreover, I have noted that this way of understanding inviolability accords with the intuition that if, in a supreme emergency, some innocent persons may be sacrificed to save a great many, the choice should be blind to differences in excellence or worth or capacity for well-being among persons—that inviolability requires every person to have a fair chance of avoiding the sacrifice or, to put the same point negatively, that all should be equally liable to being sacrificed.[21]

Nevertheless, although I believe that the threshold understanding of inviolability sketched above is the correct one, I do not pretend to have demonstrated that this is so. Instead, I will settle for a more modest conclusion: at least on one plausible understanding of the view that personhood confers inviolability, namely, the threshold view, the emergence of postpersons (assuming we can make sense of that idea) would not in itself diminish the moral status of persons, if we assume that moral status is itself a threshold concept, distinct from the concept of a gradient of moral considerability. This modest conclusion has an important implications, however: even if enhancement produced beings that were as cognitively and motivationally superior to us as we are to rats, it would not follow from this inequality alone that they would have a higher moral status. That would only follow if the inviolability of persons were not a threshold concept. According to the threshold concept of inviolability, the reason that persons are inviolable and rats are not is *not* that persons have *greater* cognitive and motivational capacities than rats and consequently "higher" interests; it is that persons have the cognitive and motivational capacities that confer inviolability and rats do not. On this view, moral status is not a matter of relative superiority; it is a matter of sufficiency. That is what it is to understand moral status as a threshold concept.

To argue persuasively that biomedical enhancements could create beings for whose sake (mere) persons could be permissibly sacrificed, one would have to do one of two things. One would either have to supply what we do not now have, namely, a threshold conception of moral status different from that which contractualist moral theories assign to persons, and then argue that while ordinary, unenhanced persons do not meet that threshold, biomedical enhancements could produce beings who do; or, one would have to argue that the idea of moral status, understood as a threshold concept, ought to be abandoned in favor of the idea of a gradient of moral considerability.

Utilitarians take the latter option. For a utilitarian there are no differences in moral status properly speaking; there is only a gradation, a continuum of beings with lesser and greater capacities for well-being and harm, and sacrificing some beings for the sake of others further along the continuum is always in principle not only permissible, but even required. On this view, if biomedical enhancements produced beings with greater capacity for well-being than persons, then persons could be justifiably sacrificed for their sake. For reasons already noted, this utilitarian view is more properly characterized as a rejection of the idea of moral status than as a noncontractualist interpretation of it.

Even if it is true, as I have suggested, that the understanding of moral status that best fits our moral intuitions makes it difficult to understand how biomedical enhancements could produce beings with a moral status higher than that of persons, I do not pretend to have settled that issue conclusively here. To do so would ultimately require a convincing resolution of the dispute between Kantian and utilitarian moral theories. Instead, I will opt for a more guarded, but still significant conclusion: unless one adopts an interest-based view according to which it would be more accurate to speak of moral gradients rather than different statuses, the worry that biomedical enhancements of some but not all would create a new moral status of postperson is highly dubious. Further, the more weight one gives to the idea of moral *status*—as opposed to the idea of a continuum of moral considerability—the more difficult it is to imagine how biomedical enhancements could produce beings with a higher moral status than that of persons.

Whether we adopt an interest-based or a respect-based view makes a great deal of difference to the answer to the question, "Could biomedical enhancements eventually produce beings with a higher moral status than that of persons?" If one adopts the interest-based view, then it is hard to rule out the possibility that the answer is "yes." In contrast, from the perspective of the respect-based view the answer appears to be "no" and the very possibility of an affirmative answer seems unimaginable. I have argued that the interest-based view is not so much an account of moral status as a debunking of the notion and a proposal to replace it with the idea of variable moral considerability. If the interest-based view is correct, then we have exaggerated the moral difference between persons and animals and should replace the idea of a difference in moral status (i. e., the threshold notion) with that of a continuum of moral considerability. But if that is so, then the prospect of postpersons is not such a dramatic change as we first thought. To the extent that the interest-based view *debunks* the notion of moral status, invoking that view to support the possibility of enhanced postpersons *deflates* the claim that such beings would have a higher moral status. So, the claim that enhancements could produce postpersons turns out to be either very implausible or not nearly as interesting as it first appeared to be.

A practical worry

Even if the emergence of beings with capacities far greater than ours would not in fact diminish our moral status (where moral status is understood as a threshold concept), these enhanced beings might *think* themselves so superior that they would treat (mere) persons as if they had a lower moral status than they have. Call this the Practical Worry. George Annas warns that "... 'improved' posthumans would inevitably come to view the 'naturals' as inferior, as a subspecies of humans suitable for exploitation, slavery, and even extermination."[22]

Even if Annas's talk of "inevitability" is unwarranted, it would be a mistake to shrug off the Practical Worry as fanciful *a priori* moral psychology.[23] There is considerable evidence that human beings have been prone to make erroneous judgments about moral status and that these judgments have played a significant role in large-scale human rights violations. For example, Africans were thought by some to be less than persons—beings with a moral status akin to that of animals—and this belief may have contributed to the practice of slavery, or at least to its persistence into an era in which it was widely thought wrong to enslave human beings.[24] It may also be the case that where disparities of power are very great, the risk of making erroneous moral status judgments—or of merely ignoring the moral status of the weak in the headlong pursuit of one's own interests—is exacerbated. To paraphrase Hume, perhaps the most the unenhanced could expect of the enhanced would be pity or charity, not justice.[25] The history of racism and of our treatment of "lower animals" and mentally disabled human beings indicates that the Practical Worry is not to be taken lightly.

Putting the practical worry in perspective

Nevertheless, the prognosis may not be quite as bleak as Annas assumes, if we attend to more recent history. *Some* inroads have been made against the worst abuses of racism and *some* improvement has occurred in the treatment of persons with mental disabilities. The modern human rights movement has done *something* to help protect the world's "unenhanced" humans and to articulate the demand that they should have access to resources needed to reap the fruits of development. And although nonhuman animals are still often horribly abused, there has been progress in our treatment of them as well, in spite of the fact that they, unlike persons, cannot speak for themselves, cannot politically organize, cannot invoke the idea that they have moral status—and cannot use weapons against us. So, it is premature to conclude that, in a world in which biotechnology exacerbated the "enhancement gap" among humans, the enhanced would "inevitably" mistake or callously ignore the moral status of the unenhanced. Much would depend upon whether the enhanced were merely stronger and smarter or also were *morally* enhanced, with greater capacity for empathy, a clearer understanding of the real basis of moral status, and more impressive powers than we possess for resisting the temptation to exploit others.

The Practical Worry is extremely serious, but it is important to understand that it is a worry about the consequences of misunderstanding or ignoring moral status, not a problem that arises because our moral concepts are inadequate or will become obsolete in the face of the prospect of biomedical enhancements. Because my focus in this chapter is on the implications of biomedical enhancement for our most basic moral *concepts*, in particular, the concept of moral status and that of human rights, I will not explore the Practical Worry in any more detail here.[26]

huh???
. .

Equal Moral Status, Different Rights?[27]

So far I have argued that even if the eventual cumulative result of biomedical enhancements (perhaps in combination with evolutionary changes) was the emergence of posthumans, the concept of human rights would not thereby be rendered obsolete, and the emergence of beings with a higher moral status would not in itself diminish the moral status of (mere) persons. I have also suggested that the idea that biomedical enhancements might produce postpersons, beings with a higher moral status than that of persons, is highly dubious, unless one is willing to embrace an interest-based view that in effect replaces the idea of status, understood as a threshold concept, with that of a continuum of moral considerability. I now want to consider a more subtle issue of equality that the prospect of biomedical enhancement raises. Could the use of biotechnologies to enhance humans eventually result in a two-tiered system of rights, even if it did not produce a class of beings with a higher moral status than that of persons?[28]

Enhanced cooperators

Consider this scenario. Suppose that some but not all human beings were enhanced in such a way that they came to have much greater cognitive abilities, including a significantly augmented capacity for complex practical reasoning, higher "emotional intelligence," and much greater capacity for empathy and for impulse control. Suppose that when enough individuals came to have this package of enhancements, they became capable of much more sophisticated, more productive, and more morally admirable forms of cooperation—with each other. This scenario is not as fanciful as it first seems. In fact, it will be familiar to those acquainted with recent work in evolutionary psychology. On some accounts, one branch of hominids—our ancestors—through some fortuitous combination of genetic change and cultural innovation, achieved a somewhat less robust package of just such enhancements, perhaps as recently as 100,000 years ago on some estimates.[29] As a result of these enhancements, large-scale, stable cooperation became possible; some might even say that morality became possible.

The troubling future scenario is one in which not all become enhanced cooperators, but so many do that what might be called *the dominant cooperative framework* is profoundly transformed: the mainstream economy and the most important political processes are structured for enhanced cooperators. The result is that the unenhanced in effect become disabled: they are unable to participate, or unable to participate in a minimally competent way, in core economic and political processes that are designed for beings with quite different capacities.

The idea of a dominant cooperative framework requires careful elaboration. Although we often speak of "the" economy, this is an idealization: there are sub-economies of various sizes, domains of production and exchange that sustain some people, even if they are quite limited in scope and less sophisticated in their forms of interaction than the mainstream economy and are somewhat independent of it. For example, a small rural village could be said to have a subsistence-cum-barter economy, even if it is embedded in a country that is increasingly integrated into a more complex, industrialized global economy that operates through currency exchanges and credit, not barter, and in which most production is for exchange, not consumption by the producer. Similarly, a person who is unable to participate in national political processes might still have considerable scope for political participation at the local level. Yet in the modern world, political processes at the national level have a profound influence on peoples' lives, and those political processes tend to focus on the mainstream economy. Because how well the vast majority of people fare depends upon the mainstream economy, there is a point to talking about "the economy" even if this is shorthand for "the mainstream economy."

The mainstream economy and the most important political processes interact to such an extent that together they may be called the dominant cooperative framework. The most important political processes take as one of their primary objects the management of the mainstream economy, and the mainstream economy generates patterns of wealth distribution that influence the character of the most important political processes. The cooperative framework that is constituted by the interaction of the mainstream economy and the most important political processes is aptly called "dominant" because, at least where it is highly developed, it is likely to operate in ways that systematically disadvantage other forms of economic and political activity.

If the gap between the enhanced and the unenhanced were great enough, the unenhanced would not be able to participate at all in the mainstream economy or the most important political processes or both. They would be like young children who, although capable of playing the extremely simple card game, "Go Fish," are unable to play Bridge and find themselves in a venue in which the Bridge players are able to determine what game will be played. Of an ordinary 3-year-old, we do not say that she is unable to play Bridge well or effectively; we say she is unable to play Bridge.

If the gap between the enhanced and the unenhanced were not so great, the unenhanced might be able to participate to some extent, but not in a minimally competent way. To grasp the implications of such a scenario, the card game analogy is again useful. Suppose there is a group of people, all of whom want to play cards. Suppose that half the group is capable of playing Bridge, but the other half can only play the child's game "Go Fish." If the group tries to play Bridge, then the game will be spoiled for those who can play Bridge, because the Go Fish types will mess up the play. If the group plays Go Fish, all can play effectively (because virtually no skill is required), but those who could play Bridge will lose a lot of enjoyment. Suppose also that the Bridge types do not stand in some special relationship to the Go Fish types that obliges them to ignore their own interests in playing a more rewarding game. In these circumstances, there is a conflict of legitimate interests. On the one hand, there is the interest of the Go Fish types in being included in the game. On the other hand, there is the interest of the Bridge types in playing a game that allows the exercise of their skills and makes possible the goods that come from the complex competition and cooperation that Bridge involves. Of course, this conflict of legitimate interests could be resolved if the group is allowed to split into two: one to play Bridge, the other to play "Go Fish." This will not be possible, however, if there is only one deck of cards.

If a large majority of biomedically enhanced cooperators come to shape the mainstream economy and the most important political processes in their own image, as it were, then the situation will be analogous to that in which there is only one deck of cards. The functioning of the dominant cooperative framework will make it increasingly hard for unenhanced cooperation to thrive—unless the enhanced cooperators opt for a dominant cooperative framework that is far from suitable, from their perspective. Where "cooperators" and "enhanced cooperators" occupy the same cooperative space—where it is impossible or very costly to avoid interactions that can be disruptive to their respective forms of cooperation—there can be a conflict of legitimate interests.

The situation I am describing is not fanciful. It exists in every complex society: there are some individuals, now called "people with developmental disabilities," who cannot function as well in complex social cooperation as "normal" people.[30] The legal rights of such individuals are restricted. Depending upon the degree of their mental or emotional impairment, they may not be able to enter into contracts, vote, marry, or hold certain kinds of jobs. The standard justification for these restrictions is paternalistic: we are protecting the developmentally disabled from injuring themselves or being exploited. However, as the card game analogy suggests, there is another, nonpaternalistic justification: some restrictions on the participation of "simple cooperators" in complex cooperation may be justified from the standpoint of a just accommodation of the conflicting interests of the "complex cooperators."

Simple cooperators have legitimate interests in being effective participants in their society's dominant cooperative scheme, where this includes the interest in not being stigmatized as incompetent to participate, and not being regarded as dependent beings who do not contribute to social cooperation. Complex cooperators have a legitimate interest in being able to engage in forms of cooperation that allow for the exercise and development of their skills, and an interest in the fruits of the greater productivity that complex cooperation can bring. The conflict of legitimate interests may be mitigated to some extent if the simple cooperators could be assured that (a) complex cooperation will produce goods that cannot be gotten through simple cooperation and that (b) they, the simple cooperators, will in fact have adequate access to these goods. But it would be wrong to *assume* that such goods would fully compensate for the simple cooperators' exclusion from participation in the dominant cooperative scheme and the stigmatization that this typically involves.

Beyond a certain point, getting more of the goods that can be made available to them through the participation of others in the dominant cooperative scheme may be less important to the unenhanced than being able themselves to participate in the cooperative scheme. A conflict of legitimate interests may remain even if sincere efforts to compensate the unenhanced are undertaken.

The extent of the conflict may be mitigated if the individuals involved do not evaluate alternative cooperative schemes exclusively on the basis of how well they facilitate the satisfaction of their own preferences. They may value inclusiveness in its own right. Honoring the commitment to inclusiveness may require a mutual sacrifice of legitimate interests. Similarly, even if individuals value inclusiveness, the question remains as to how much weight this value ought to be accorded. So, the assumption that the enhanced, the unenhanced, or both have moral commitments regarding cooperation does not eliminate the conflict of legitimate interests. If a more demanding cooperative framework is chosen, the unenhanced will lose something they rightly value; if a less demanding one is chosen, the enhanced will lose something they rightly value.

Equally legitimate interests, unequal rights

If both groups continue to operate in the same cooperative space, then just accommodation of these conflicting legitimate interests may require that *both* groups settle for something less than their first choice as to what the dominant cooperative scheme will be like, if they only took into account the satisfaction of their own preferences (considerations of justice or inclusiveness aside). The complex cooperators—the enhanced—might have to settle for a less demanding (and less rewarding) cooperative framework than they are capable of participating in effectively; and at the very least they would have to compensate the simple cooperators for any restrictions on their participation, and in such a way as to acknowledge the costs of stigmatization and dependency that the simple cooperators would suffer. The simple cooperators might have to settle for some restrictions on their participation in the more demanding areas of the dominant cooperative framework. It is perhaps worth noting that the Americans with Disabilities Act—perhaps the most comprehensive existing attempt to avoid discrimination against persons with disabilities—tacitly acknowledges that justice requires *mutual* accommodation, *not* the maximal promotion of the interests of persons with disabilities. It requires only "reasonable accommodation" of the special needs of persons with disabilities; it does not require that society make *whatever* changes are necessary, regardless of the losses to nondisabled people, in order to remove all impediments to full participation on the part of those with disabilities.[31]

There is an important difference, however, between the sorts of compromises regarding the cooperative framework that might be required to accommodate the legitimate interests of unenhanced cooperators in our thought experiment and the modifications of the existing cooperative framework that are typically demanded by people with disabilities. When people with disabilities demand ramps for wheelchairs or Braille panels in elevators, they are asking for changes that will give them access to the existing cooperative framework, but that do not make that framework any less suitable for the nondisabled. Unenhanced cooperators are not like short adults who need a higher chair to be able to reach the Bridge table; they are like 3-year-olds who cannot play Bridge. To make it possible for the unenhanced to be effective participants, it might be necessary to "dumb down" the cooperative framework itself, thereby making it less valuable for the enhanced cooperators.[32]

Suppose, then, that biotechnologies were used to develop a series of enhancements that eventually resulted in the emergence of a large group of enhanced cooperators, but that some remained unenhanced. Suppose that the new form of cooperation of which the enhanced cooperators were capable was not only more materially productive and much more rewarding to them than simpler forms of cooperation, but also was more morally admirable in the sense that it cultivated higher levels of moral virtues in the participants and facilitated more morally praiseworthy achievements and relationships. If enhanced and unenhanced cooperators competed for the same cooperative space, then there might be a conflict of legitimate interests. A just accommodation of the conflicting legitimate interests might require some differences between the rights of the enhanced and unenhanced. The enhanced might have a range of rights that allow them participation in areas of the dominant cooperative scheme that are off-limits to the unenhanced. Both groups might enjoy the same *basic* rights, but the enhanced would have a richer set of rights in addition.

Notice that nothing in this scenario suggests that the unenhanced would have a higher moral status. The conflict of interest is between two different groups of persons. But even if we need not worry about biotechnologies producing beings with a higher moral status, we ought to consider the possibility that they might produce a two-tiered system of rights. The idea of a two-tiered system of rights is not novel, of course; I have already noted that it is exemplified in the legal system's treatment of people with developmental disabilities. At least from the standpoint of an understanding of rights that acknowledges that claims about their existence require justifications that appeal ultimately to the legitimate interests of persons, we must be willing to consider the possibility that a just accommodation of the conflicting interests of enhanced and un- enhanced cooperators may involve different moral rights, not just dif- ferent legal rights. The prospect that the pursuit of enhancements may proliferate inequalities in rights is troubling.

Equal moral status, different rights?

Beings with the same moral status can have different rights, but only within limits, because the idea of moral status, at least in the case of persons, is intimately connected with the idea of rights. Indeed, as I noted earlier, the moral status of persons is typically explicated in significant part *in terms of rights*: persons as such are said to have certain basic moral rights. All persons having certain basic rights in common is compatible with their having different rights from one another, so long as the different rights are not basic rights. However, the distinction between the basic rights that help define moral status and other, nonba- sic rights may be difficult to draw and is certainly a contested matter in moral theory. We may need a clearer notion of moral status than we now possess to be able to draw a plausible distinction between basic and nonbasic rights. Or we may need to develop better theories of rights to clarify our concept of moral status.

Is a hierarchy of rights compatible with public recognition of equality?

Whatever else is true about the moral status of persons, this much seems clear: proper acknowledgment of a person's moral status requires some sort of fundamental *public recognition of equality.*[33] But surely a commitment to the public recognition of the equality of persons places significant constraints on inequalities in the rights of persons, if only for the reason that human beings with inferior rights may find it hard to regard themselves—and harder to be regarded by others—as having equal moral status. The Practical Worry returns, in a more sophisticated form.

So, the concern that enhancement could actually produce beings with a higher moral status and the Practical Worry that enhanced beings would act as if they possessed a higher moral status, even if they didn't, are not as crisply distinct as first appears. The commitment to equal moral status, if it is to be sincere and realistic, must take into account the facts, including the facts of moral psychology, that determine the conditions under which the ideal of equal moral status can be realized.

Equal political participation rights and equal moral status

Daniel Wikler suggests that the cognitively enhanced might reasonably conclude that the unenhanced were not fit to manage their own affairs.[34] He concludes that an unequal distribution of civil liberties would be justified. He does not consider whether unequal civil liberties are compatible with proper recognition of equal moral status. The more interesting question, in my judgment, concerns political participation rights, because, at least on some views, they are more intimately connected with equal moral status. Could a large, enhanced majority justifiably deny political participation rights to the unenhanced?

Jeremy Waldron has argued that, at least in the mainstream of liberal political thought, the struggle for equal political participation rights is based on the idea of equal status.[35] According to Waldron, Locke's view (at least when it is purged of sexist and racist distortions) is that the same capacity for rational self-direction that confers a distinctive, higher moral status when compared with nonrational beings, also qualifies one for equal participation in governance. On this view, it is highly problematic, if not outright inconsistent, to assert that enhanced cooperators would not be of a higher moral status even though they had fundamental rights of political participation that the unenhanced did not possess.

Quite apart from the question of whether moral status and political participation rights are as intimately connected as Locke suggests, there is good reason to be skeptical about the claim that biomedical enhancements could justify the denial of political participation rights to the unenhanced. Consider the form that an argument for restricting political participation rights to the enhanced would take. The idea would be that only the enhanced should have political participation rights because only they can properly understand the complex workings of society or have the moral capacity to work for the common good in a consistent and farsighted way.

There are two points to notice about this argument. First, it is a very old one. Plato advanced it in *The Republic*. It is simply the argument that only the most intelligent (or the most intelligent and virtuous) are fit to rule. Second, whether this argument (or some refinement of it) is cogent does not depend upon how those with superior characteristics came to have them, so envisioning the possibility of biomedical enhancements seems to add nothing that can help us determine whether it is cogent.[36]

The objections to the Platonic argument are so well known that it is not necessary to rehearse them all here. Instead, I will only mention two of the most prominent. The first is that even very considerable differences in intelligence and virtue do not qualify the superior to rule over others without their participation in governance because such an arrangement is too risky for the nonparticipating: their interests are not likely to be adequately represented. The second is that the value of political participation is not purely instrumental. Thus the less intelligent have a stake in political participation even if their participating makes government less efficient.

To argue convincingly that biomedical enhancement could justify unequal political rights one would have to do one of two things: successfully defend the general form of the Platonic argument against the well-known objections to it; or show that a proposal for unequal distribution of political rights between the biomedically enhanced and the unenhanced would be immune to those objections. Neither option looks promising, in my judgment. The well-known objections seem cogent and seem to apply with equal force to the biomedical enhancement version of the Platonic argument, unless one can adequately defend the very problematic assumption that the instrumental value to those who would lack political participation rights would be so great as to overwhelm the noninstrumental value of participation. Here a quite different analogy than that of the card game may be apt: suppose that human affairs could be run much more efficiently if God were to micromanage them, eliminating the need for human governance entirely. It is far from obvious that this gain in efficiency would justify the claim that human beings have no right to govern themselves. What is more, imagining a scenario in which biomedical enhancements elevate human beings to anything approaching the wisdom and beneficence attributed to the deity may be even more difficult than the task we confronted earlier, that of imagining how biomedical enhancements could create postpersons.

Conclusion

I've argued that if biomedical enhancements produced a sharp division between simple cooperators and complex cooperators, the result could be that individuals with the same moral status would have different rights (so long as these do not include the "basic" rights that equal moral status entails). Thus, even if the prospect of biomedical enhancements does not challenge the assumption that all who qualify as persons have the same moral status (the Equal Moral Status assumption) or render the concept of human rights obsolete, it may nevertheless pose a serious threat to equality. So, a moral assessment of the pursuit of biomedical enhancement technologies ought to take seriously the risk of this sort of inequality. In the next and final chapter I advance a proposal for institutional change that would help reduce this risk.[37]

Notes

1. Expressing this worry, Francis Fukuyama suggests that, "The ultimate question raised by biotechnology is, What will happen . . . once we are able to, in effect, breed some people with saddles on their backs, and others with boots and spurs?" See Francis Fukuyama (2002), *Our Posthuman Future* (New York: Farrar, Straus and Giroux), pp. 9–10. As stated, this statement is ambiguous. It could mean that some people will actually have a lower status, or that they would be simply treated as if they did. I will consider both alternatives in this chapter, but will focus on the former. Jeff McMahan

also considers the possibility that enhancement could produce beings with a higher moral status than persons in "Cognitive Enhancement and Moral Status" (unpublished paper). Daniel Wikler explores the possibility that, if some but not all were sufficiently cognitively enhanced, it might be justifiable for the enhanced to restrict the legal rights of the unenhanced. He does not frame his discussion in terms of different moral statuses, but as I argue below, it is directly relevant to that issue. Daniel I. Wikler (2009), "Paternalism in the Age of Cognitive Enhancement: Do Civil Liberties Presuppose Roughly Equal Mental Ability?" in *Human Enhancement*, Julian Savulescu and Nick Bostrom (eds.) (Oxford: Oxford University Press), pp. 341–55.

2. In what follows, I examine both Kantian and Utilitarian conceptions of moral status, in an effort to make sense of the worry that enhancement might produce beings with a higher moral status. It might be said that in doing so I have failed to consider two alternative sources of concern. The first is the idea, present in some variants of the Christian tradition, of a "great chain of being," created by God, with human beings at the top, placed there in a position of rightful dominance over the rest of creation. On this view, for humans to create beings who were "higher" than human beings would be to act contrary to God's design and would presumably be wrong for that reason. There is a familiar ambiguity in this view: are humans entitled to dominate lesser creation simply because God willed that those who were at the top of the great chain of being should dominate, or did God will that we should dominate because it is fitting that those with "higher" capacities should dominate those with lower ones? The latter alternative points toward a second view, reasonably attributed to Nietzsche, expressible in non-theological terms: those who have superior (more evolved or developed or complex?) capacities are entitled to dominate. I will not consider the theological view here, not only because those bioethicists who voice the worry about enhancement producing unequal moral statuses insist that they are not relying on theological premises, but also because I think the descriptive idea of a great chain of being, and along with it the notion that nature is teleological in any way relevant to morality, has been irrevocably discredited by evolutionary science. I will engage the Nietzschean view to this extent: I will argue that the most familiar and plausible view of moral status rules out the claim that greater strength or power, or even virtue, itself entitles one to a higher status. At this point I will only say that the Nietzschean view seems either to confuse the possession of a rather arbitrarily constricted set of individual excellences with basic moral worth, or to be committed to the utterly implausible claim that power grounds right, that the more powerful are entitled to more because they are more powerful.

3. See, for example, Allen Buchanan (2004), *Justice, Legitimacy, and Self-Determination: Moral Foundations for International Law* (Oxford: Oxford University Press), especially Chapter 3.

4. See, for example, Francis Fukuyama (2003), *Our Posthuman Future: Consequences of the Biotechnology Revolution* (Profile Books); and Erik Parens (1995), "The Goodness of Fragility: On the Prospect of Genetic Technologies Aimed at the Enhancement of Human Capacities," *Kennedy Institute Journal of Ethics* 5: 141–153.
5. I thank Janet Radcliffe-Richards for clarifying this point.
6. Jeff McMahan, "Cognitive Enhancement and Moral Status" (unpublished paper); Daniel Wikler (2009), "Paternalism in the Age of Cognitive Enhancement: Do Civil Liberties Presuppose Roughly Equal Mental Ability?" in *Human Enhancement*, Nick Bostrom and Julian Savulescu (eds.) (Oxford: Oxford University Press).
7. See Leon Kass, "The Wisdom of Repugnance" (2000), in *The Human Cloning Debate,* 2nd edn., Glenn McGee (ed.) (Berkeley, CA: Berkeley Hills Books), pp. 68–106; Fukuyama 2002, supra note 1.
8. Norman Daniels (2009), "Can anyone really be talking about ethically modifying human nature?" in *Enhancement of Human Beings,* Julian Savulescu and Nick Bostrom (eds.) (Oxford: Oxford University Press) pp. 25–42.
9. My concern here is not to defend this conception of human rights, but to plumb its implications for the prospect of biomedical enhancements. For a systematic critique of it, see Charles R. Beitz (2009), *The Idea of Human Rights* (Oxford: Oxford University Press).
10. Indeed, if "humanity" refers to the class of persons, it does not even imply that the concept of human rights applies to all human beings in the biological sense, since not all of these are persons.
11. Most secular theories of human rights agree that human rights are grounded in the interests or capabilities that (normal) human beings have, but some theories hold that a sound justification for the ascription of human rights to individuals requires premises that refer not only to individuals' capabilities or interests, but also to facts about institutions. Nothing in these theories requires that only human beings have the interests or capabilities in question.
12. As indicated in note 2, their concern may have another source: they may have tacit religious beliefs or strongly teleological beliefs of a nonreligious sort to the effect that there is a natural order and that the creation of beings with a higher moral status than humans (or persons) would destroy or disturb it. For a critique of this type of view, see Allen Buchanan (2009),"Human Nature and Enhancement" *Bioethics* 23(3): 141–150.
13. See Stephen Darwall (2006), The Second-Person Standpoint: Morality, Respect, and Accountability (Harvard University Press).
14. This description of "development as enhancement" is compatible of course with a recognition that the processes of development involve losses as well as gains and in no way implies that people in less developed countries are

inferior people. See Allen Buchanan (2009), "Human Enhancement and Human Development," *Kennedy Institute of Ethics Journal* 18: 1–34.

15. This formulation is intended to be broad enough to cover the distinction Jeff McMahan makes between interests and time-relative interests. McMahan, *The Ethics of Killing: Problems at the Margins of Life* (Oxford: Oxford University Press), pp. 232–242.

16. This notion of mutual accountability encompasses a range of broadly contractualist views, including those of Darwall and Scanlon. See Darwall 2006, supra note 13; T.M. Scanlon (1998), *What We Owe to Each Other* (Cambridge, MA: The Belknap Press of Harvard University Press). On such views it is the capacity to engage in certain kinds of *relationships* that counts, but these can rightly be described as capacities nonetheless.

17. Although I believe there is much to be said for the view that interest-based conceptions are implausible because they are committed to the view that talk of the moral status of persons is a misleading way of talking about the special importance of certain kinds of interests, nothing I say in the remainder of this chapter depends on that being the case.

18. This objection was raised by Jeff McMahan at a conference on Enhancement and Human Nature, in Hong Kong, December 7, 2007.

19. The notion of inviolability at issue here is one that limits inviolability to beings that have rights. Ronald Dworkin develops a different conception of inviolability that is not limited in this way. He uses "inviolability" and "sacredness" interchangeably, although he does not invoke the religious connotations of the latter. According to Dworkin, something (including inanimate objects such as great works of art) can have inviolability because of the creativity involved in their histories. Because I am concerned here with notions of inviolability that are spelled out in terms of rights, I will not pursue Dworkin's discussion further.

20. I thank Jeff McMahan for pressing this objection also.

21. Of course, the claim that differences in capacities for well-being should not determine who is to be sacrificed means here only that having *relatively* greater capacity should not count. This is compatible with requiring that those who are to be eligible, in a fair lottery, for being saved through the sacrifice of others, must be capable of *significantly* benefiting from being saved.

22. George Annas (2005), "Cell Division," *Boston Globe*, April 21. See also George Annas (2005), *American Bioethics: Crossing Human Rights and Health Law Boundaries* (Oxford: Oxford University Press), p. 51.

23. For a perceptive and sensible effort to throw cold water on Annas's confident predictions of "genetic genocide" perpetrated by the enhanced on the unenhanced and a clear articulation of the point that Annas has utterly discounted the widespread benefits that enhancement could bring, see Elizabeth Fenton and John D. Arras (2010), "Bioethics and Human

Rights: Curb Your Enthusiasm," *Cambridge Quarterly of Health Care Ethics* 19: 127–133.

24. The hypothesis that mistakes about the moral status of Africans contributed to slavery is compatible with the hypothesis that the practice of slavery—more specifically, the interests it served and generated—helped foster and sustain those very mistakes.

25. "Were there a species of creatures, intermingled with men, which, though rational, were possessed of such inferior strength, both of body and mind, that they were incapable of all resistance, and could never, upon the highest provocation, make us feel the effects of their resentment; the necessary consequence, I think, is, that we should be bound, by the laws of humanity, to give gentle usage to these creatures, but should not, properly speaking, lie under any restraint of justice with regard to them, nor could they possess any right or property, exclusive of such arbitrary lords. Our intercourse with them could not be called society, which supposes a degree of equality; but absolute command on the one side, and servile obedience on the other." See David Hume (1983), *An Enquiry Concerning the Principles of Morals*, 1777 edn., J. B. Schneewind (ed.) (Indianapolis, IN: Hackett), Section III, part I, p. 25.

26. A plausible response to the Practical Worry would require two things: an adequate characterization of both the risks of enhancement (including the risk that the enhanced would wrongly treat the unenhanced as inferiors) and the benefits of enhancement, as well as a consideration of how fairly or unfairly the benefits are likely to be distributed.

27. I am grateful to Daniel I. Wikler for pressing me to consider this question in this chapter.

28. The discussion that follows draws on my reflections in Chapter 7 of Allen Buchanan, Dan Brock, Norman Daniels, and Daniel Wikler (2001), *From Chance to Choice: Genetics and Justice* (Cambridge: Cambridge University Press).

29. See, for example, Spencer Wells (2002), *The Journey of Man: A Genetic Odyssey* (Princeton, NJ: Princeton University Press), pp. 84–88.

30. See Daniel I. Wikler (1979), "Paternalism and the Mildly Retarded," *Philosophy & Public Affairs* 9: 377–392.

31. The Americans with Disabilities Act of 1990, in Section 12111(9), requires "reasonable accommodation," for example, on the part of employers but limits this requirement by "undue hardship," defined as "an action requiring significant difficulty or expense." See (9) and (10) of Section 12111 at http://www.ada.gov/pubs/ada.htm (Accessed 10 June 2010).

32. I thank John Arras for this point.

33. Elizabeth Anderson emphasizes this recognitional aspect of equality repeatedly when she argues that egalitarian justice's "proper positive aim is not to ensure that everyone gets what they morally deserve, but to create a community in which people stand in relations of equality to others." See

Elizabeth Anderson (1999), "What Is the Point of Equality?" *Ethics* 109: 287–337, at pp. 288–289.

34. Wikler 2009, supra note 1.
35. Jeremy Waldron (2002), God, Locke, and Equality: Christian Foundations in Locke's Political Thought (Cambridge: Cambridge University Press).
36. I am indebted to an Editor of *Philosophy & Public Affairs* for this important point.
37. I would like to thank Tom Douglas, Jeff McMahan, Russell Powell, Janet Radcliffe-Richards, and the Editors of *Philosophy & Public Affairs* for helpful comments on an earlier version of this chapter.

CHAPTER EIGHT

Distributive Justice and the
Diffusion of Innovations

Much has been written about the potential of biomedical enhancements to worsen distributive injustices. Some have gone so far as to advocate refraining from enhancements in order to avoid such injustices. In Chapter Two, I argued that there has been an unfortunate tendency to treat the case of biomedical enhancements as if it were *sui generis* and morally novel. I argued that enhancement is nothing new and that we should explore the ethics of biomedical enhancements through the lens of the ethics of development. Once we look at matters in this way, it is clear the mere fact that some might lack access to valuable enhancements cannot in itself be a sufficient reason to refrain from creating them, anymore than the mere fact that some now lack access to modern healthcare systems, the rule of law or literacy means that no one should enjoy these benefits. Seeing biomedical enhancement through the lens of the ethics of development also helps us avoid another, equally serious error: smugly assuming that the benefits of biomedical enhancements will "trickle down" to the worst off. Even if valuable innovations tend to become more widely available over time, they may do so too slowly.

In a world in which innovation is a central fact of life, the diffusion of beneficial technologies should occupy center stage in our thinking about distributive justice. My suggestion is that we approach the problem of injustices in the distribution of valuable biomedical enhancement technologies by recognizing that it is only one aspect of the larger problem of injustices resulting from the inadequate diffusion of technologies.

A caveat is in order. I am not assuming either that all enhancements are beneficial or that when they are beneficial their wider diffusion is always a good thing. Instead, I am focusing on cases where the lack of access to highly valuable enhancements results in injustices. The first step in thinking productively about this particular problem is to situate it within the larger issue of justice in innovation.

Justice in a world of innovation

Contemporary theorists of distributive justice do not make the mistake of thinking that the problem of justice is that of fairly dividing a fixed stock of goods. They acknowledge that what is available to distribute changes as our productive capacities develop, that what is produced and how much is produced are subject, within constraints, to choices that human beings make, and that these choices should be guided by principles of justice. To that extent, their views are at least *consistent* with a remarkable fact about modern society: the prominence of innovation in our lives, especially in the form of new technologies developed through the application of scientific knowledge. Yet the significance of innovation for justice—the opportunities for promoting justice it creates, and the risks of injustice that it poses—has not been adequately appreciated by theorists of justice.[1]

In "Toward a theory of justice in innovation," I first explain why a theory of justice must take the fact of innovation seriously and then focus on one important problem of justice in innovation: the fact that when powerful innovations do not diffuse widely, but are available only to some, this creates opportunities for domination and exclusion, as well as the loss of opportunities for improving the well-being of the world's worst off people. In "The Global Institute for Justice in Innovation," I advance a proposal, developed in collaboration with Robert O. Keohane and Anthony Cole, for a Global Institute for Justice in Innovation (GIJI), a new international institution designed to ameliorate this problem. The reader should be prepared for a kind of gear-shifting in the exposition of this book at that point. The GIJI proposal is very concrete and detailed, in keeping with one of the major themes of this volume, namely, that at this point in the enhancement debate, what is needed is policy proposals for coping with the challenges of enhancement that are definite enough to be of some practical use, not an endless iteration of the pros and cons of enhancement. "The Status of the GIJI under International Law" explains how the GIJI could be integrated into existing international law.[2] This section also is quite detailed, but if we are to go beyond vague gestures toward something of practical value, specificity is needed.

The GIJI is designed to promote justice in innovation in general, not just innovations that are used for biomedical enhancements. Focusing exclusively on the problem of the diffusion of biomedical enhancements or even of enhancements generally would be arbitrary. Problems of justice arise, not because a valuable innovation is an enhancement or because it is a biomedical enhancement, but because some lack access to it and their lack of access deprives them of benefits they are entitled to or makes them vulnerable to domination, exploitation, or unfair competitive disadvantage.

I concluded the preceding chapter with the sober thought that if some lack access to biomedical enhancements, they might be excluded from full participation in the dominant cooperative framework of their society. In this chapter I consider realistic measures that could be taken to avoid this outcome.

My aim in this chapter is not to make a conclusive case for creating the new institution I describe. It is to demonstrate the value of situating worries about injustice in the distribution of biomedical enhancements in the larger context of an institutional approach to the problem of justice in the diffusion of innovations. More generally, I want to show what it is like to take the idea of an institutional response to the challenges of enhancement seriously. This chapter will also help to flesh out further the idea of the enhancement enterprise. To embark on the enhancement enterprise is, *inter alia*, to develop institutional resources for coping with the ethical issues that enhancement raises, including problems of justice.

Toward a Theory of Justice in Innovation

The need for an account of justice in innovation

Innovation is significant from the standpoint of justice because it can have either positive or negative effects on justice. Depending on what is created and to whom it becomes available, innovation can worsen existing injustices or create new injustices, or it can lessen existing injustices.

Justice in innovation is not restricted to the just distribution of *existing* beneficial innovations for two reasons. First, as the much-discussed case of essential medicines makes clear, the fact that vitally important innovations are *not* occurring can be a concern of justice, at least according to some theories of justice. If the medical research agenda for the most effective pharmaceutical companies is determined largely by market demand and the political influence of disease advocacy groups in the developed countries in which these companies are based, then medicines that could save the lives of millions of people in less developed countries, at relatively low cost, may not be developed. (Research dollars may flow to the development of hair loss remedies and super-Viagra and not to the development treatments or vaccines for malaria or dysentery—to name only two of the worst killers in the less developed world.) On some understandings of justice, including those that include a human right to healthcare (even of a rather limited sort), this situation is not just unfortunate, but unjust. Second, if powerful innovations are available only to some, this may contribute to injustices of other sorts, even if the fact that some lack access to the innovation is not itself an injustice. This would be the case if restricted access to the innovation resulted in unjust inequalities of political power or in other forms of wrongful domination. History is replete with instances of this scenario. Think of the role which unequal access to technologies played in the worst depredations of colonialism, for an example.

Given these possibilities, it is clear that taking the fact of innovation seriously in theorizing about justice requires more than including the products of innovation—the new things that actually happen to get produced—among the goods that are directly subject to principles of just distribution. Justice may also require efforts to shape the innovation process: to influence which innovations will occur, either to prevent innovations that would worsen existing injustices or create new injustices, or to encourage innovations that would lessen existing injustices. Accordingly, we can define "justice in innovation" as the conformity of both the distribution of the fruits of the processes of innovation, and of the character of the innovation process itself, to the requirements of justice.

The fruits of innovation, like other socially produced goods, should themselves be distributed in conformity with the requirements of justice, but the impact of innovations on the distribution of *other* goods is also subject to the requirements of justice. Furthermore, justice in innovation may require a pro-active stance. It may not suffice to wait and see what innovations come about and then try to deal with their impact on justice *ex post*; rather, it may be necessary to shape the innovation process in the name of justice, either to try to avoid the production of justice-degrading new technologies or to harness the innovation process for the purpose of promoting justice.

How innovation can promote justice

To the extent that thinking about justice has focused on innovation, concern about the negative impact of innovation on justice has been prevalent. Some of the most powerful enhancements, including genetic modification of embryos, neural tissue implants, and brain–computer interface technologies, are likely to be expensive. The worry is that they will be affordable, at least at first, only to the better off and that this will exacerbate existing injustices.[3] Similarly, "the digital divide"—the fact that some people lack access to computers—can itself contribute to political and social inequality and may also exacerbate existing injustices in the distribution of other goods, including wealth.

Less attention has been given to the potential of innovation generally and of biomedical enhancements in particular for *promoting justice*. To correct this imbalance, consider the following examples of technological innovations that may have significant justice-*promoting* effects. In each case the innovation in question could be seen as promoting justice by reducing unjust advantages that some people enjoy or by empowering individuals so that they can more effectively exercise their rights.

1. Some cognitive enhancement drugs are most efficacious for the less bright; to the extent that existing social arrangements unfairly disadvantage those with lower intelligence or lower intelligence results in part from socio-economic injustices, making such drugs available to the latter could be justice promoting.[4] Such pharmaceutical cognitive enhancements might prove more cost-effective than some educational interventions.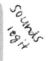

2. Cheap calculators help "level the playing field" for those who are mathematically challenged, thus reducing injustices that may arise from the ways in which society rewards those with math skills, or penalizes those who lack them.

3. Medical innovations can remove disabilities that interfere with opportunities individuals ought to have as a matter of justice or that prevent them from exercising their rights.

4. Computers allow small businesses to reduce costs of marketing, identify low-price inputs, manage distribution, etc., and thereby can help reduce unjust barriers to entry into markets dominated by large companies.

5. Cell phones allow cheap, rapid coordination of economic and political activities; this can help people to lift themselves out of poverty and enable them to exercise their rights of political participation more effectively.

6. Internet access to medical information reduces knowledge asymmetries between physicians and patients and this in turn can reduce the risk that patients' rights will be violated.

7. Cell phone cameras provide checks on police behavior, thus helping to reduce violations of civil and political rights or at least facilitate remedial action when they occur.

The point is that while some innovations worsen injustices, others may ameliorate them. Whether an innovation is justice damaging or justice promoting will depend not only on the characteristics of the innovation, but also on the social context in which it is deployed. Once again, sweeping generalizations are to be avoided.

Disagreement and uncertainty about justice

Each of the preceding seven innovations appears to reduce certain *inequalities*, but not all inequalities are *injustices*. To know which inequalities are unjust, and hence whether particular innovations are impacting justice positively or negatively, one needs an account of justice. Theorizing about justice is notoriously afflicted, however, with both disagreement and uncertainty. There are disagreements between consequentalists and deontologists, between proponents of "positive" rights and libertarians who acknowledge only "negative" rights, between egalitarians, prioritarians, and sufficientarians, and among egalitarians as to what the "currency" of egalitarian justice is (well-being, opportunity for well-being, or resources). There is also uncertainty as to how to move from a given theory's abstract, highest-level principles to lower-level principles with clearer implications for policies and institutions. For example, even if one assumes one knows what the proper principles of distributive justice are for what Rawls calls the basic structure of society, it is not clear which principles of justice should guide particular policies or decisions about rationing scarce medical resources.[5] Given that there is no indication that this disagreement and uncertainty is likely to be resolved in the foreseeable future—how should thinking about justice in innovation proceed? How *can* it proceed in a principled way?

A provisional starting-point: the injustice of extreme deprivation.

Most theories of justice converge on the belief that what might be called extreme deprivation is presumptively unjust, at least when it is undeserved and unchosen. "Extreme deprivation" can be understood in different ways, but the idea is perhaps best initially conveyed by examples: people suffer extreme deprivation when they lack adequate food, shelter, safe drinking water, are afflicted with serious preventable diseases, and when their physical security is seriously compromised by the threat of violence, as in the case of civilians in war zones. Alternatively, it may be useful to think of extreme deprivations as those severe harms that basic human rights provide protections against.[6]

A commonsense proposal is to proceed on the assumption that whatever else it should be concerned with, a theory of justice in innovation should treat extreme deprivation as a matter of concern, in two ways: it should provide guidance both for reducing the risk that innovations will produce or exacerbate extreme deprivations and for helping to ensure that the power to innovate will be harnessed to help ameliorate existing extreme deprivations. The practical strategy, then, would be to consider policies regarding innovation that would address the concern about extreme deprivation, without waiting for a resolution of the disagreement and uncertainty that characterize current theorizing about justice. Even if there is disagreement or uncertainty about the inclusion of some particular harms under the rubric "extreme deprivations," surely there is enough agreement that some harms should be included to allow us begin to grapple with the problem of justice in innovation.

Exclusion and domination

To focus *only* on extreme deprivation, however, is too restrictive, for reasons already indicated: it overlooks the fact that innovation can be a concern of justice when the fact that some but not all have access to innovations results in unjust exclusion or domination. The analogy with disabilities rights shows that unjust exclusion can occur without severe deprivation and that these are distinct injustices. Even if a person with mobility limitations is not impoverished and leads an otherwise comfortable life, she may rightly complain of injustice if she is barred from access to public buildings.

Extreme inequalities in political influence can result in extreme deprivation or at least can contribute to its continuation. But political inequalities need not result in extreme deprivation to be unjust. The fact that women in the US lacked the right to vote until 1920 was an injustice, apart from whatever contribution it made to the extreme deprivation that some women suffered. Similarly, if some innovation in electronic communications conferred advantages in influencing national political processes, in ways that are incompatible with the commitment to broad effective political participation embodied in democratic institutions, this would be an injustice, even if those who lacked access to the innovation in question suffered no extreme deprivation.

Some inequalities in political power are inevitable even in the most democratic societies; and some inequalities in political power are not unjust, including those that result from special excellence in the qualities of political leadership. But under modern conditions, in which the State wields such great power over our lives, inequalities in political power have the potential to exacerbate existing injustices and undermine justice where it exists.[7] So political inequality is a proper *concern* of justice even if the people involved are integrated into the society and political inequality is not in itself unjust.[8]

For the purposes of this chapter, it is not necessary to take a stand on the issue of whether political inequalities are only a matter of concern for instrumental reasons or also because they threaten the public affirmation of fundamental equality. It is enough to note that both instrumental considerations grounded in the strategic nature of political inequalities and views according to which political equality is valuable in itself converge on the conclusion that political inequalities are a proper concern of justice, independently of their propensity to create or sustain extreme deprivation.

For convenience and brevity, I will use the phrase "basic political and economic inequalities," to refer, not to just any unequal distribution, but only to (a) seriously unjust inequalities in political power and (b) lack of access to important sites and forms of social cooperation that is of comparable consequence to the exclusion suffered by persons with disabilities in societies that do not take disability rights seriously. My suggestion is that an account of justice in innovation should not be limited to a concern about extreme deprivation, but should also address the potential impact of innovation on "basic political and economic inequalities" understood in this way.

It could be argued that the impact of innovation on extreme deprivations is a higher priority, from the standpoint of justice, than the impact on basic economic and political inequality. Whether or not that is so may depend upon the resolution of deep disputes in the theory of justice—in particular whether some form of prioritarianism, some special emphasis on the needs of the worst off, is the correct view. I have already explained why I think it is appropriate to avoid attempts to resolve such disputes before embarking on an attempt to develop a principled practical response to the issues of justice in innovation.

From the standpoint of many persons in developing countries, the main concern about innovation is its potential positive or negative impact on extreme deprivation, but for most of those who live in developed countries the impact on social and political inequality may be more pressing. Given that this is so, there are two reasons to include basic economic and political inequality, not just deprivation, in our provisional conception of justice in innovation. First, it is a *legitimate* concern for people generally, regardless of whether they live in developed or developing countries, even if deprivation is the more serious moral concern. Second, practical thinking about justice in innovation must take the problem of political feasibility seriously, and generally that requires engaging the interests of the better off. An approach to justice in innovation that focuses not only on deprivation but also on basic social and political inequalities is more likely to gain wider support and, crucially, the support of those who are critical for its success.

The threads of the argument thus far can now be pulled together. Because of the prominence of innovation in modern life, thinking about justice should take seriously the potential of innovations both to worsen injustices and to ameliorate them. Given pervasive disagreement and uncertainty about what justice requires, a reasonable approach for the present would be to focus initially on the least controversial injustice—

undeserved and unchosen severe deprivation. This narrow focus needs to be expanded, however, to encompass "basic political and economic inequalities"—seriously unjust inequalities in political power and exclusion from the most important sites and forms of productive cooperation. Biomedical enhancements *might* turn out to be among the innovations that have the greatest potential impact on justice understood in this way, but there is no reason to think that they will be unique in this regard.

Types of institutional strategies

There are three basic types of institutional strategies for the pursuit of justice in innovation: (1) *prohibition* of innovations that would worsen existing injustices or create new injustices; (2) *creation* of innovations to ameliorate existing injustices; and (3) *diffusion* of innovations in order to avoid injustices that would arise from differential access to them or to promote justice by ameliorating or removing existing unjust disadvantages.

Prohibition

Voluntary abstention from the development and diffusion of valuable innovations would likely fail because of familiar free-rider and assurance problems.[9] In addition, voluntary restraint would be in tension with the scientific ethos of discovery, except perhaps where scientists believed that a potential innovation would clearly have a preponderance of unambiguously bad uses or consequences. Regulation (coercively backed prohibitions) to try to stop development and/or diffusion of innovations thought to have unjust inequality-increasing effects is hardly more promising, for at least two reasons. First, the innovation process is by its nature highly unpredictable and the effects of an innovation on justice, whether for good or for ill, may be especially hard to predict. Consequently, a coercively backed prohibition strategy might deprive us of valuable innovations that would turn out to be consistent with the demands of justice or which might even promote justice. Second, and more importantly, if a certain line of research and development is prohibited in one country or regional governance regime (such as the European Union), it is likely to be taken up in less regulated locales, as has happened across a wide range of cases, including gene therapy and human embryonic stem cell research. For a number of reasons, including the lack of regulatory capacity in many countries, an effective, worldwide scheme of regulatory prohibition, while conceivable in principle, is unlikely in the foreseeable future.

Creation

There are many examples of private and government efforts to spur innovations of various sorts: research grants, government contracts, and public and private prizes being among the most obvious. Few of these efforts to stimulate innovation are explicitly directed toward issues of justice in innovation. One exception to this general tendency is the US Orphan Drug Act, which provides research grants and extended patent life for drugs developed to treat serious diseases that afflict small numbers of people. One plausible interpretation of the purpose of this legislation is that it is designed to ameliorate the unfairness of a situation in which the direction of drug research and development is determined by market demand rather than need, to the life-threatening disadvantage of those with rare diseases. Several more recent proposals to ameliorate the "essential medicines problem" can also be seen as efforts to stimulate the creation of drugs for the purpose of promoting injustice.

Diffusion

Limited or slow diffusion of a beneficial innovation can be problematic from the standpoint of justice for either or both of two reasons: once created, innovations do not mitigate problems of inequality unless they are diffused widely to the disadvantaged; and if diffusion is too limited or occurs too slowly it may actually produce new injustices, either by giving unacceptable advantages in political power to those who do have access to them or by excluding those who lack access to them from important sites or forms of economic cooperation. For convenience, I will use the term "the diffusion problem" to refer to both of these phenomena. In the preceding chapter, I explained how biomedical enhancements, especially cognitive enhancements that enabled new more complex forms of cooperation, might be subject to the diffusion problem.

A wide range of existing programs, projects, and organizations exemplify the strategy of promoting the diffusion of technologies in order to avoid or mitigate injustices due to lack of access or to promote justice by removing existing unjust disadvantages. An illustrative list might include the following:

1. Private and government efforts to bridge the "digital divide" by providing subsidized or free computers, high-speed and/or wireless internet service, etc.

2. Private and government programs designed to diffuse more widely the extremely valuable cognitive enhancement technology commonly known as literacy.

3. Vaccine delivery programs in less developed countries, where infectious diseases are still a major contributor to childhood mortality.

4. Donation or reduced pricing of "essential medicines" through arrangements between governments and pharmaceutical companies (in particular, antiretroviral HIV/AIDS medications).

5. Private provision of financial/economic technologies to the poor, for instance through NGO-provided microfinancing.

6. "Compulsory Licensing," as recognized by the World Trade Organization (WTO)'s Doha Declaration on trade-related aspects of intellectual property rights (TRIPS) and Public Health, which acknowledges the right of States to grant licenses for producing essential medicines without the permission of intellectual property rights (IPR) holders, if certain standards are met.

These examples of diffusion promotion policies are not part of an overall strategy, formulated in response to the articulation of goals of justice in innovation. Instead, they reflect an uncoordinated, piecemeal approach and they have not addressed biomedical enhancements. In the next section, I outline a systematic proposal for promoting justice in innovation that emphasizes diffusion strategies and proceeds on the basis of a realistic appraisal of international institutional capacity. The core of this proposal is a new institution—GIJI. The proposal also does something to address the Creation Problem, but its main focus and distinctive contribution concerns the Diffusion Problem. More specifically, the proposal addresses one important impediment to diffusion: the monopoly pricing that results from the current IPR regime.[10] Insofar as diffusion that is inadequate from the standpoint of justice results from the current IPR regime, it can be regarded as an institutional failure. The core idea of the proposal is to modify the IPR regime in a way that preserves its valuable functions while remedying or at least significantly ameliorating this failure.

The Global Institute for Justice in Innovation

The GIJI would be an international organization designed to construct and implement a set of rules and policies governing the diffusion of innovations on the basis of a sound set of principles. It would operate under conditions of accountability, according to rule-governed procedures, and would seek gradually to inculcate norms that specified appropriate behavior with respect to the diffusion of innovations.[11] The GIJI would be created by a multilateral treaty, with permanent staff, and international legal authority to make decisions that were not automatically incorporated into the domestic law of its member States, but only became enforceable as a result of political and constitutional processes by each member State. In this sense, the GIJI would be similar to the WTO, the rules of which are directly effective only on the international level, rather than the European Union, which requires as a condition of membership that certain rules be directly applicable in domestic legal proceedings. Such an arrangement would limit the sovereignty costs of the GIJI.

A subsidiary activity of the GIJI would be to encourage the creation of useful innovations, for example through prizes and grants for justice-promoting innovations, and through offering extended patent life for innovations that have a positive impact on justice, as with the Orphan Drug Act. But its major efforts would be directed toward the wider and faster diffusion of innovations in order to ameliorate extreme deprivations and reduce their negative impact on basic political and economic inequalities, as defined above. As noted earlier, the focus would not be restricted to biomedical enhancements, but if biomedical enhancements became a prominent instance of the problem of justice in diffusion, the GIJI would allocate its energies accordingly.

The GIJI would actively promote diffusion entrepreneurship, that is, efforts by NGOs and others to accelerate the diffusion of justice-promoting innovations. Its most important asset, however, would be a "licensing option," under which the GIJI would obtain the right to authorize compulsory licensing on a country-by-country basis of innovations that are diffusing too slowly. "Too slowly" here means that the innovations are failing to realize their potential for making significant gains in promoting justice, or are exacerbating existing injustices, in the form of extreme deprivation or basic political and economic inequalities. Member governments of the GIJI would enact legislation authorizing the relevant domestic authorities to initiate administrative actions to issue compulsory licenses for intellectual property that has not diffused as fast as a published set of guidelines specifies. Since the proposal to allow centrally directed compulsory licensing of intellectual property in these cases is, to our knowledge, a new idea, I will focus on it in what follows.

The licensing option

Member states would enact laws authorizing domestic patent authorities to grant compulsory licenses to firms or other entities selected by the GIJI free of charge or for nominal fees. Licenses would be distributed so as to create a competitive market, thereby reducing the price of the innovation to competitive levels. Thus, if the current slow diffusion of the product is due to monopoly pricing, freely distributing the license would accelerate diffusion. Some innovations, however, diffuse slowly because they are of little value. This is why the GIJI would have a licensing *option*. It would only act where there is evidence that the obstacle to diffusion would be removed by authorizing compulsory licenses and creating a competitive market for the innovation in question.

It is important to understand the political implications of the GIJI's authorization option. Without imposing supranational authority over governments, such authorization would render mandatory licensing by a developing country internationally legitimate. In view of the broadly representative nature of the authorizing body, to be discussed in more detail below, it would be hard for companies, in such a situation, to claim unfairness. The GIJI would therefore greatly strengthen the bargaining position of countries that had well-founded claims of insufficient diffusion. As noted below, it would also protect firms against attempts by opportunistic governments to abuse compulsory licensing to seize private property. This proposal, therefore, does not try to suppress or avoid politics (a quixotic venture in international relations) but to shape politics in desirable ways.

If the GIJI's threat to authorize mandatory licensing has sufficient credibility, and imposes sufficiently high threat of loss on the firm, exercise of the GIJI licensing option should be a rare event. The threat of mandatory licensing would deter producers from exercising the capacity for monopoly pricing that IPRs confer. Producers would know that they can keep their full IPR by refraining from monopoly pricing in the case of innovations whose slow diffusion would have a negative impact on justice. The GIJI would monitor the diffusion of justice-impacting innovations and issue public warnings of possible licensing unless diffusion increased by some minimal magnitude within a certain time period. Producers would know that they could avoid the negative publicity of being warned about mandatory licensing, and could receive public praise and reward (through the prizes and grants policy), if they act in ways that promote justice. Over time, this array of incentives could help foster the norm of taking justice into account in the innovation process.

Stages of intervention

Exercising the licensing option would be a last resort, to be used rarely if at all. The GIJI would construct a "watchlist" of innovations that warrant scrutiny from the standpoint of inadequate diffusion. Producers of innovations on the watchlist would be notified, without public announcement, that they are on it and that if diffusion does not improve, a *publicized* warning of potential liability to mandatory licensing will be issued in due course. If there were no significant improvement or evidence of significant efforts on the part of the producer to bring about improvement, the GIJI would initiate its internal process for authorizing mandatory licensing and announce that it was doing so. Such authorizations would be both (1) time-limited and (2) area-specific. Compulsory licensing would be authorized for a limited time period only, say from one to as much as 10 years, depending upon projections as to how long it would take to achieve a significant increase in diffusion, and the time required for the licensee to receive an adequate return on its initial investment. If the diffusion problem was limited to certain less developed countries in which access to the innovation is critical (as is the case with medicines to combat malaria, for example), then the innovator would lose IPRs only with respect to that area market.

After the GIJI had authorized compulsory licensing, there would be another period in which the firm whose products were under scrutiny could change its policies to promote diffusion, giving another opportunity for compromise before mandatory licensing was imposed.

Since this proposal allows ample room for negotiations and adjustment of policies, it is necessary to consider the likelihood that firms and States supporting them might use this opportunity not to adjust their own policies but instead put pressure on weaker States not to exercise their authority to invoke compulsory licensing. To reduce this risk, several measures would be necessary. There would have to be a clear legislative statement of observable "pressuring" actions that were inappropriate in conjunction with a GIJI process for compulsory licensing, and of the period of time in which they were inappropriate (any time after the GIJI started considering compulsory licensing for a given product in a given country). Inappropriate actions would include any actions that would be reasonably interpreted as a punishment or threat toward a country that utilized a GIJI authorization for compulsory licensing. Such actions would include (*inter alia*): withdrawing products from a country's market or raising prices/royalties on them, or threatening to do so, unless it is part of a general policy applying to a set of similar countries; threatening the withdrawal of other forms of international aid, or withdrawal of support on an unrelated issue in another forum. On a complaint by a State against a company or another State, a GIJI process would be set in motion involving conciliation, an arbitral panel, and the GIJI's Appellate Tribunal, as necessary.

If a State or company were found responsible for such actions, it would be put on probation. Complaints against companies or States on probation would be put on a fast track, bypassing the conciliation stage and shortening time periods for each stage in the process, while nonetheless remaining within the limits of due process. Lists of States and companies on probation would be published, and penalties for repeat offenses would be steeply increased. Such a process would strongly discourage coercive interference with a State's decision to utilize the GIJI's authorization of compulsory licensing, while not violating due process or mixing judicial with legislative functions.

Given that compulsory licensing would be time-limited and area-specific, and that the option need rarely be exercised for its purpose to be realized, this proposal can be properly characterized as a modification of existing IPR, not a radical overturning of them.

Compensation

A crucial question involved in designing the GIJI concerns policies toward compensation to IPR holders for the acquisition of authority to issue licenses to others to produce their products. At one extreme of a continuum, one could imagine a policy providing no compensation. Such a policy would have the advantage of deterring monopolistic practices and would enable the Institute to operate on a relatively small budget. But there are three decisive objections to a no-compensation policy. First, innovation would be discouraged, especially innovations designed to help poor people in poor countries, since it is precisely these innovations that would be subject to GIJI authorization of compulsory licensing. Second, significant alterations would be necessary to many contemporary international agreements, including TRIPS and numerous bilateral investment treaties, which require that some level of compensation be paid upon the compulsory licensing of a patent. Third, it is virtually unimaginable that such a policy would be endorsed by wealthy countries that are home to the most innovative firms in such fields as pharmaceuticals and electronics, and whose ratification of a Treaty for Justice in Innovation would be essential for the GIJI to have a meaningful impact.

At the opposite extreme of this continuum would be a policy calling for full market-value compensation. Such a policy would not significantly discourage innovation, if it were credible that full market-value compensation would remain the Institute's policy. Furthermore, providing full market-value compensation could have the advantage of making it more likely that rich, powerful countries would support creation of the Institute. However, if a full market-value compensation policy were to be adopted, it would essentially use public funds to pay monopolistic prices to private firms. Such a policy would be unpopular with democratic publics, and it would be difficult to raise sufficient sums to finance many such licenses. Furthermore, it would not deter monopolistic behavior—it might even encourage it.

It seems clear that neither zero compensation nor compensation at the full (monopolistic) market value of the innovation is satisfactory. Hence some middle ground will have to be found. A "fair price," representing a substantial but not exorbitant rate of return for the company, would have to be paid. In our view, current theorizing about justice does not ground a unique determination of a "fair price" here; instead, there is probably a range of reasonable alternatives. One of the first actions of the GIJI would be to devise a set of procedures through which a fair price would be determined, and administrative law procedures providing for notice and comment and review by the judicial arm of the GIJI, as discussed in the section on accountability below. The trick is to pick a pricing system that creates the right incentives, given the goals the licensing option is designed to promote, and avoids any clear unfairness to any of the parties concerned. Since anything less than paying the monopoly price could somewhat discourage innovation, the GIJI might find that its diffusion strategy would be more effective if combined with subsidies for the creation of promising innovations, compensating for the speculative but sometimes alluring prospect of very large monopolistic profits in the long run.

Compensation would be paid directly by the GIJI, rather than through the traditional approach of the payment of royalties from sales of licensed products, in order to avoid the price increases that would result from royalties. Such an approach would be consistent with the GIJI's goal of increasing diffusion of innovations, as a lower price would maximize the number of individuals able to afford the innovation in question.

Political decision-making by the GIJI

One of the major functions of the GIJI would be to assess the justice implications of the pace at which useful innovations, including biomedical enhancements, were diffusing to disadvantaged people, either those suffering severe deprivation or those laboring under burdens of basic economic and political inequalities. Carrying out this function would be contentious and large amounts of money could be at stake, so the GIJI's decision-making arrangements would need to be carefully designed. What follows is only a sketch of one possible design, in the interests of promoting discussion.

The GIJI would have an administrative unit with the competence to analyze relevant information about diffusion and its effects, and the authority to propose exercise of the Institute's licensing options and other actions. The model here is something between the Secretariats of the WTO, which is relatively small and definitely subordinate to the organization's membership, and the World Bank or the International Monetary Fund, which are operated by a much larger administrative organization that makes many decisions with only general supervision from its Board. The Executive Head of the GIJI could not order licensing of IPR on her own, but could propose licensing to an Assembly of the GIJI.

The Assembly, which would meet annually, would have a tripartite composition roughly modeled on the International Labor Organization. Its members would include representatives of states, NGOs with substantial records of service to disadvantaged people (such as Save the Children and Oxfam), and firms holding patents.

The problem of credentialing NGOs for participation in the Assembly warrants careful attention, but is not insoluble. The same issues arise with respect to the roles of NGOs in other international institutions. In addition to having a public commitment to addressing diffusion issues and experience in or at least directly relevant to the performance of this function, participating NGOs would have to satisfy familiar requirements of transparency, financial integrity, independence from governments and corporate interests, and responsiveness to the preferences and needs of those individuals and groups they claim to represent or on whose behalf they claim to act.

Each of the three constituencies would elect its representatives at the Assembly. As in the Montreal Protocol Fund, governments of developed and developing countries would have equal numbers of representatives, elected separately from these constituency groups. For the sake of concreteness, consider one possibility: there would be an Assembly of 32 representatives, consisting of eight industrialized countries, eight developing countries, eight NGOs, and eight innovation-producing firms. It is important that the numbers not be too large; the Montreal Protocol Fund body, with fourteen members, has operated very well, much better than the unwieldy universal bodies involved in the Kyoto Protocol and post-Kyoto negotiations. Important decisions in the Assembly would require a form of supermajority voting designed to ensure that decisions had wide support, although it would be equally important to avoid a veto by any group.

Decisions by the GIJI Assembly to authorize compulsory licensing would require a supermajority for immediate action, coupled with a majority of the votes in three of the four categories of representatives. Demanding immediate action, NGOs and developing countries could not join with one or two industrialized countries to exercise a licensing option; on the contrary, they would have to get a majority of either industrialized countries or firms. There could be a provision for relaxing this requirement after a delay (say, of 1 year) in order to give IPR holders and others time to voice disagreement. After this waiting and discussion period, the requirement could be relaxed to, say, a majority of votes in three of four categories or 60 percent of the votes overall. The idea is to promote deliberation and compromise, but not to give any one group (such as major drug companies supported by the United States) a veto.

These procedures seem suitable for the kind of decision that authorized licensing represents. Licensing important intellectual property rights would be a major decision, with very significant financial and political implications that extend over a long period of time. By necessity, it would be controversial. Most important, in a desirable equilibrium such a decision would never be finalized. Instead, the prospect of authorized licensing could deter monopolistic practices that would unduly retard diffusion of justice-impacting innovations.

The GIJI would begin with informal warnings about the pace of diffusion, followed if necessary by formal public proposals for notice and comment. These measures could threaten sufficiently serious reputational harm to the company involved that it would be prompted to take measures to accelerate diffusion. A really successful GIJI would never mandate any compulsory licensing, but would provide incentives for firms to diffuse the fruits of their innovations more quickly. Indeed, the GIJI could give awards or prizes to firms that had consistently exceeded its diffusion standards, thus providing the firms with reputational benefits.[12]

The successful operation of this new institution would depend on the following functions being performed by it or by other institutions whose activities were coordinated with it.

1. *Research* to identify, sponsor, integrate and make available the best information on patterns in the emergence and diffusion of technologies from the standpoint of their impact on justice: which

technologies, under which conditions, for how long, either increase or decrease extreme deprivation and basic political and economic inequalities. (This would include, for example, research to identify which sorts of design features increase the opportunities for accelerating diffusion of valuable innovations by "piggy-backing" the on pre-existing, widely-diffused technologies.)

2. *Surveillance* to develop "early warning" and information sharing about the justice impact of innovations.

3. Identification and dissemination of *best practices* among private and public entities concerned to promote justice in innovation. One of the most important functions of the GIJI would be to encourage other institutions and organizations to help perform these three functions and to provide a forum for organizing an efficient institutional division of labor to achieve them. As the only international institution devoted to addressing issues of justice in innovation, it could serve an important coordinating function for a variety of other institutional and organizational efforts. In this connection, it would develop a sophisticated website as a global clearinghouse for information on the diffusion of innovation. Indeed, the existence of such a prominent website could heighten attention worldwide to issues of innovation justice, and could in the end be even more important than its authority to acquire intellectual property rights.

Accountability

The basic structure and key procedures of the GIJI would be deliberately designed to promote accountability. The composition of the GIJI Assembly would ensure that the organization is accountable, not just to the States that ratify the treaty which creates it—both with developed and developing economies—but also to various publics whose interests are represented by NGOs, and to the community of innovators. Furthermore, accountability would be enhanced by the stipulation that all major organizational actions, including acquisitions and changes in operating rules, are subject to administrative due process.

Proposals to authorize compulsory licensing could only be made under a set of rigorous due process requirements. First, the Executive Head of the GIJI would have to make a public announcement of intention to propose compulsory licensing of a specific set of intellectual property rights in a specific country for a specified period of time, and the GIJI would have to provide clear means for comments and discussion. This procedure would be similar to the "notice and comment" procedures of US administrative law, which require Federal agencies to publish potential rules, allow time and opportunity for interested parties to complain and make suggestions, and require a reasoned response from the agency proposing the rules. After the required period of perhaps 45 or 60 days had elapsed, the GIJI would have to re-issue its proposed order for compulsory licensing, at which point it would formally be put on the docket of the Assembly. Decisions of the GIJI could be reviewed for conformity to due process standards by an Appellate Tribunal, roughly modeled on the Appellate Body of the WTO.[13] That is, there would be a public set of procedures that encouraged compromise but provided for rulings by expert panels that could be appealed to the Appellate Tribunal, composed of judges selected for relatively long terms. The Appellate Tribunal would hear cases in public and issue public decisions providing reasons, which could serve as precedents to develop a body of GIJI law.

Funding

The GIJI's funding would come chiefly from member States, on a sliding scale, according to ability to pay. On the model of the World Bank subscription system,[14] countries would commit funds as necessary in large amounts—funds that would be essential for ensuring IPR holders that were subjected to compulsory licensing received fair compensation.[15] Traditionally, compulsory licensing compensation has come from royalties paid by licensees of the IPR in question. In contrast, direct payment of compensation from the GIJI would mean that compensation rates could be set by the GIJI at a fair level, rather than just at the likely significantly lower level necessary to ensure the product remained affordable to the poorest consumers in the market. Having these funds readily available would be essential for the credibility of the GIJI's warnings that it was intending to order compulsory licensing. Indeed, with the resources essential to assure credibility at hand, the GIJI's authority to license IPR would operate mainly as a deterrent to monopolistic pricing. Insofar as the deterrent was effective, the funds might never need to be drawn upon. In addition, if the GIJI gained sufficient prestige, private donors might find it attractive to help fund the organization's grant and prize activities.

Is the proposal a morally unacceptable modification of existing IPRs?

It might be objected that the GIJI's ability to authorize compulsory licensing is based on a flawed assumption, namely, that innovators are morally responsible for injustices that result from inadequate diffusion of their products. This is not the case: there is no assumption that innovators have any special moral obligation to promote justice through the diffusion of their products. The proposal is for modifying the existing *legal* IPR regime in such a way as to remedy or at least ameliorate one of its negative consequences: inadequate diffusion due to monopoly pricing. Of course the proposal for modification is based on moral assumptions, but so is the case for the existing IPR regime. The reasons for modifying the existing IPR regime in the way we suggest are chiefly moral, but they do not include any such assumption about the moral responsibilities of innovators.

The existing IPR regime should not be viewed as a legal embodiment of a supposed "natural right" to property on the part of creators of valuable things. Instead, as reflected in the existence of compulsory licensing provisions under contemporary domestic intellectual property laws, it is most plausibly seen as an instrument for serving a plurality of values that includes not only a proper recognition of the value of creativity and the distinctive relationship that may exist between the creator and her creation, but also the promotion of social welfare and considerations of justice. All of these values would be relevant considerations in designing an IPR regime from scratch, and all are relevant to evaluating and possibly modifying the existing regime. An IPR regime that exclusively promoted any one of these values to the detriment of the others would be indefensible. This is true even in the case of distributive justice: an IPR regime that systematically thwarted opportunities for massive gains in aggregate welfare out of fastidiousness for avoiding relatively trivial injustices in the distribution of welfare would be unacceptable. (It is one thing to say that the mere fact that a policy would increase aggregate welfare is not a reason for doing what is unjust, but quite another to say that no gain in aggregate welfare, no matter how great, can ever justify a departure from the strict requirements of justice.)

Similarly, even if an IPR regime should bestow special legal entitlements on creators, this moral consideration must be balanced against other moral considerations, including the avoidance of serious inequalities in political power.

The GIJI's ability to order compulsory licensing does not assume that innovators have any special moral obligations regarding distributive justice; it only assumes that whatever moral rights innovators have regarding their creations, this does not rule out the very limited form of interference with existing legal IPRs that properly exercised compulsory licensing entails. My surmise is that any theory of innovators' "natural" moral rights that would make these rights robust enough to rule out the GIJI's authorization of mandatory compulsory licensing would not only be implausible in its own right, because it would give short shrift to other relevant moral values such as distributive justice and the promotion of social welfare, but would also be hard to square with the restrictions on innovator's rights that that the existing IPR regime already includes.

At any rate, this proposal is directed toward those who view the existing IPR regime as roughly within the bounds of the reasonable and the morally acceptable, not toward radical natural rights views that ascribe extremely broad, indefeasible "natural" moral rights to innovators. Moreover, the argument is *comparative*: given a reasonable construal of the existing IPR regime as an instrument designed to serve a plurality of widely held values, our proposed modification of it does a better job of balancing those values. It ameliorates a very troubling side-effect of monopoly pricing without an unacceptable decrease in incentives for innovation.

Is the proposal politically realistic?

One could expect the GIJI to be greeted with at least cautious enthusiasm by developing countries and NGOs. Of course, their bargaining strategies will temper their public support, since they will be working for more favorable terms; but in fact they have much to gain and little to lose from the proposal. The proposal will not be as attractive to powerful developed states and the innovation-creating firms based in these states. If the GIJI is to work, it will require the support of these States, including especially the United States and Japan, and the European

Union, and at least acceptance by major firms—which might itself be a necessary condition for support by powerful States. If adequate support depended upon altruistic motivations of the sort that are rarely exhibited in the behavior of States, this would be a serious strike against the proposal. So, the pertinent question is this: Without making unrealistic assumptions of altruism, what incentives would powerful States have to help create and to sustain the GIJI?

Before identifying the positive incentives, it is important to note that the GIJI does *not* threaten the constitutional sovereignty of States: that is, their legal supremacy and independence.[16] States would retain their ability to make final decisions on issues of importance to them. While it is proposed that developing countries in particular structure their domestic laws to facilitate giving effect to GIJI decisions to authorize compulsory licensing, all member States would retain the ability to determine for themselves how much control to deliver to the GIJI, and would also retain the right to decide whether to take up any authorizations they received. The GIJI's rulings would not have direct effect within domestic jurisdictions, and could not override domestic laws. Moreover, there would be a provision in the GIJI statute enabling States to withdraw from the organization, with due notice.

Like the WTO, the GIJI would constitute an *exercise* of sovereignty by States, limiting in some ways their own legal freedom of action. Members of the GIJI would be publicly committed not to thwart the purposes and actions of the organization—for instance, by threatening retaliation against the GIJI for ordering compulsory licensing of IPR owned by their own firms, if these acquisitions were judged by the Appellate Body to have been carried out in conformity with its rules and procedures. In this sense, the treaty underlying the GIJI, like all international legal agreements, would limit the legal freedom of action of States.

There are four major positive reasons for developed countries and their firms to support the GIJI. The first and most general is that more rapid diffusion of innovations would accelerate economic development worldwide—a long-term goal of developed countries, as it is in their interests to enhance both prosperity and the chances for a peaceful and more democratic world order. Wide diffusion of innovations would create conditions facilitating the creation of more innovations in more diverse ways, some of which would almost certainly rebound to the advantage of people in developed countries.

Unfortunately, appeals to general interests are often not persuasive to either firms or governments. The next three reasons for developed countries and their firms to support the GIJI are more specific. Reason number two—perhaps the most persuasive to innovative firms and their governments—is that the GIJI's role in evaluating patents for potential compulsory licensing would directly address concerns that producers and developed countries have with the current WTO-sanctioned compulsory licensing procedures. While presently IPR holders remain vulnerable to compulsory licensing decisions by domestic authorities at times driven by domestic political pressures, decisions at the GIJI would be reached within a system in which both developed countries and IPR producers themselves are active participants. Developing countries would, of course, retain the power to order compulsory licenses without sanction by the GIJI. However, any decision to order a compulsory license that either had previously been rejected by the GIJI or was never submitted to the GIJI would be difficult to defend in the public arena, and inconsistent with claims that it was being pursued for the public good.

The third and fourth reasons are both reputational. The GIJI would provide significant reputational advantages to IPR holders involved in disputes about alleged monopolistic pricing that harms disadvantaged people. At present, these disputes take place in an open public sphere, in which interest groups with the best soundbites and the media play a large role. Major drug companies were quite bruised, for example, by the campaigns against them at the beginning of the millennium with respect to pricing of AIDS drugs—campaigns that often portrayed the companies as rapacious profit-seekers unconcerned about the welfare of poor AIDS sufferers in Africa. The GIJI would give the companies and their supporters a forum for their own defense: if a GIJI that was regarded as legitimate by attentive world publics ruled in favor of the company, this would provide compelling support for its reputation.

The fourth reason concerns the reputations of countries rather than firms: by supporting a new institution designed to promote fairness as well as development, the developed countries would be making a powerful symbolic statement at relatively low cost to themselves. The reputation of the rich countries for being willing to help poor ones has been badly damaged by their reneging on promises in the Uruguay Round of trade negotiations (1987–94) to reduce trade barriers to agricultural products. While the various agricultural lobbies in rich countries may make fulfillment of those pledges impossible, moving ahead with the GIJI could demonstrate good faith. It is too much to hope that financially powerful companies involved in innovation would enthusiastically support this proposal for an institution that could mandate licensing of their intellectual property. But their grudging acceptance of the GIJI would certainly facilitate its operation. The GIJI is designed to minimize threat to these firms. It could reward innovators with prizes, grants, and extended patent life. Any licensing decisions would result in companies being compensated at fair value, even if at a lower rate than monopolistic pricing would provide. As noted above, companies that met the GIJI standards for adequate diffusion of their innovations—i.e., those that were not singled out for possible acquisition—would be able to cite this fact to defend themselves against charges that they were engaging in unfair, monopolistic practices or being overly aggressive in marketing their products.

There is no denying that the GIJI would be a "hard sell" for drug companies and other patent-holders whose business plans count on monopolistic returns on successful innovations to compensate them for huge up-front investments, many of which yield no commercial products. However, the ability of the GIJI to authorize licensing on a national basis, rather than globally, would mean that patent-holders would retain their IPR in countries in which diffusion was indeed adequate, these being the countries in which current revenue from the innovation in question would predominantly come. Nonetheless, in most cases their home governments would have to decide, in response to public pressure and foreign policy incentives, to support the GIJI proposal and to induce or force their companies to acquiesce. Public pressure and attention to the problem of innovation diffusion, in industrialized democracies, would be essential for this proposal to gain sufficient traction to be politically feasible. But in the end, this is a modest proposal that would not fundamentally disrupt the activities of innovation-creating companies, and that might induce them to devise ways to accelerate diffusion of their innovations in ways that rebounded to their long-term benefit.

The problem of diffusion of innovations is much broader than the problem of lack of availability of essential medicines to the poor. Many innovations that could have an important impact on justice are *not* like anti-malarial drugs: access to them will be beneficial not just to those in less-developed countries but to virtually everyone, and the problem they present for justice is not that they are unlikely to be produced by the market. This is perhaps especially likely to be true of biomedical enhancements, as opposed to treatments of diseases. Consider, for example, biomedical technologies that extend years of vigorous life or that augment the immune system, or drugs that enhance important cognitive skills. The difficulty here is not that there is insufficient market demand to stimulate research and development; rather, it is the risk that these valuable innovations will not be available except to the better-off or, more realistically, that they will not become available to most people quickly enough to avoid significant injustices. Even if the GIJI does not address the Creation Problem, it can make a major contribution by addressing the Diffusion Problem. From the standpoint of biomedical enhancements, the Diffusion Problem appears to be the major concern.

The Status of the GIJI under International Law

While there are a number of international agreements that would potentially affect the GIJI's actions, attention here will be paid only to the two most important types: (1) the WTO's TRIPS Agreement, and (2) Investment treaties.

TRIPS

As a mandatory agreement for all WTO Members, TRIPS has a far-reaching global impact, and thus the degree to which the GIJI and its actions would conform to the requirement of TRIPS is extremely important. The following discussion will illustrate that a WTO Member State that grants a compulsory license as a result of a decision by the GIJI would not be in violation of its obligations under TRIPS.

While there have previously been questions raised regarding the acceptability of compulsory licensing under TRIPS, its acceptability as well as the freedom of States to decide the reason for compulsory licenses being granted was explicitly confirmed in the 2001 Doha Declaration on the TRIPS Agreement and Public Health. Moreover, while TRIPS does specify some reasons for which compulsory licenses might be granted under domestic law, these are not stated to be exclusive. Consequently, so long as compulsory licensing under the GIJI operates in a manner consistent with the constraints on compulsory licensing enunciated in TRIPS, no WTO liability would attach to any appropriate action taken in accordance with a GIJI compulsory licensing decision.

Compulsory licensing restrictions under TRIPS are predominantly found in Article 31, which lists twelve procedural standards that must be met in order for any grant of a compulsory license to be TRIPS consistent. Four of the standards are of particular relevance to the GIJI, and thus will be discussed here.

Under Article 31(a), decisions to grant a compulsory license must be made on an individualized basis. That is, licenses cannot be granted for all products of a particular type, such as "all pharmaceuticals." Rather, each individual product must be considered for compulsory licensing on its own merits. As the GIJI process specifically involves evaluation of innovations on an individualized basis, this provision clearly presents no obstacle to the GIJI.

Under Article 31(b), an attempt must be made prior to compulsory licensing to obtain authorization from the patent-holder to license the patent on reasonable commercial terms and conditions. Exceptions exist to this rule, including where a national emergency or other urgent circumstance exists. However, while in some circumstances the GIJI may indeed need to rely upon this "national emergency" exception, it will usually not be necessary. The GIJI is institutionally designed to ensure that direct discussions with patent-holders occur for a reasonable time prior to any decision to order a compulsory license. Consequently, unless a "national emergency" makes a rapid compulsory licensing order necessary, the requirements of Article 31(b) will be met—and if a "national emergency" has occurred, Article 31(b) will not be applicable.

Under Article 31(h) the patent-holder must receive "adequate remuneration" to compensate it for any losses due to the compulsory license. While there is no clear agreement regarding the meaning of "adequate" as used in this provision, the goal of the GIJI to pay "fair" compensation, at a rate higher than the 2–5 percent royalty rate conventional in compulsory licensing, would seem to ensure that the compensation paid by the GIJI will indeed be more than "adequate."

Under Articles 31(i) and (j), the compulsory licensing decision must be subject to review by an authority superior to the body making the original decision. While appeals may not be available within the domestic legal system in which compulsory licensing was ordered, this requirement is clearly met by the incorporation within the GIJI of an Appellate Tribunal.

The GIJI, then, is designed in a manner that would make enactment of its compulsory licensing decisions consistent with the TRIPS obligations of the GIJI Member State concerned. Ideally, to remove any doubt, this would be reflected through the enactment of a special amendment to TRIPS clarifying that no grant of a compulsory license taken in accordance with a GIJI decision could give rise to a claim for violation of WTO obligations. However, even if such an amendment were not able to be passed at the WTO, an additional protection exists for developing countries enacting GIJI-ordered compulsory licenses, in the form of the dispute settlement system of the WTO.

As TRIPS is a WTO text, any claim that a State was in violation of its TRIPS obligations in enacting a GIJI-ordered compulsory license would have to be resolved through State-to-State arbitration, rather than through individual patent-holders directly bringing a claim against the GIJI Member State in question. However, Members of the GIJI will find it politically enormously difficult to justify bringing a WTO case against a State that has merely implemented a GIJI decision, when the complaining State itself had previously agreed, by virtue of becoming a Member of the GIJI, that the GIJI's procedures were fair. Non-Members of the GIJI would, of course, face no such obstacle. However, as already argued, there is no reason to believe that any compulsory licensing decision made by the GIJI would result in WTO liability even if a claim were brought.

Investment treaties

An enormous number of investment treaties now exist around the world, and a great number of them explicitly include reference to IPR as constituting a form of "investment." Consequently, it is possible that the granting of a compulsory license by a developing country, in accordance with a decision by the GIJI, would give rise to a claim for compensation under an investment treaty.

While investment treaties all contain a variety of grounds on which an investor can claim compensation from a State, those based on the manner in which an investment has been treated, such as "fair and equitable" treatment, would be very unlikely to serve as the basis for a claim for any action taken in accordance with a GIJI decision, due to the procedural safeguards included in the design of the GIJI. In addition, the traditional claim for "expropriation," made when a State takes the property of a foreign investor, could not be made with respect to compulsory licensing done in accordance with a GIJI decision, as the investor would retain the patent in question, but would merely be required to allow others to produce licensed versions of the product in question.

Compulsory licensing could, however, give rise to a claim of "indirect expropriation," which occurs when a State regulates an investment in a manner that leaves formal ownership of the investment with the foreign investor, but effectively takes away the benefits of the investment. While arguments would be available to any GIJI Member State forced to defend against such a claim, the unresolved nature of contemporary international investment law regarding indirect expropriation means that it is impossible to be certain that a compensable indirect expropriation would not be found.

Moreover, the structure of investment treaty dispute resolution means that the patent-holder would have the right itself to institute an arbitration in order to secure compensation for its alleged losses. Thus, unlike at the WTO, developed States would not be able simply to reject claims for compensation by their investors who have allegedly suffered losses as a result of a GIJI decision.

Nonetheless, while investors control their own claims under an investment treaty, it is important to remember that the treaty is nonetheless between the two States, with the investor having no direct roles in its implementation or interpretation. As a result, the risk of claims being raised under investment treaties as a result of a GIJI compulsory licensing decision could be significantly reduced merely by requiring States joining the GIJI to sign a declaration that no compulsory licensing granted in accordance with a GIJI decision would give rise to a claim under any investment treaty to which it was a party.[17] Alternatively, even greater protection could be gained if individual agreements were signed by GIJI Member States that were parties to investment treaties stating that compulsory licensing granted in accordance with a GIJI decision would not give rise to a claim under the specific treaty in question.

This would, of course, not be a complete solution, as claims could still be made under investment treaties involving non-GIJI Member States. Moreover, investment arbitration tribunals have recognized the right of investors to qualify as an "investor" under a specific treaty merely by undertaking the formalities of incorporation in a State party to the treaty, so long as the treaty itself permitted this. Consequently, the risk of an investment treaty claim could not be entirely eliminated by such agreements.

Nonetheless, the possibility of a compensation order being issued by an investment arbitration tribunal against a developing country due to a GIJI decision could be adequately addressed by having such claims paid by the GIJI itself where the State acted in accordance with GIJI rules and instructions. In this way, the burden would be spread amongst all GIJI Members, thus minimizing the financial burden on any individual State.

Conclusion

One of the morally unacceptable features of the contemporary world is that innovations that would be of immense value to severely deprived people, and that would ameliorate unjust economic and political inequalities, are not widely available even though the marginal costs of providing them are low. This problem could become even worse in an era of powerful biomedical enhancements. Instead of improving the condition of all human beings, biomedical enhancements might be available only to some and this disparity might worsen existing unjust inequalities or even create new ones.

One source of this problem is the patent system, which stimulates innovation by giving monopoly rights to patent-holders. Monopoly pricing by patent-holders combines with lack of resources by those who need the innovations the most to generate and sustain deprivation and inequality. The *diffusion of innovation* is blocked by the features of dominant institutions.

Since this is an institutional problem, an institutional solution is needed. The institutional solution proposed here is a GIJI. This Institute would offer prizes and other incentives for innovation, but its major task would be to promote the diffusion of existing justice-impacting innovations through a multistep process. Quiet encouragement of more rapid diffusion could be followed, when unsuccessful, with public "naming and shaming" of firms that restricted access to their products through monopoly pricing or other means. But the Institute would also have a standing compulsory licensing option for intellectual property rights whose owners were not sufficiently promoting diffusion to disadvantaged people. If informal measures did not succeed, the GIJI could authorize states to issue compulsory licenses for innovations that were not diffusing at a sufficiently rapid rate. Such proposals would have to be accepted by supermajority vote of an Assembly in which developed countries, developing countries, NGOs and firms holding intellectual property rights would be equally represented. Fair compensation, according to previously publicized procedures and guidelines, would be paid by the GIJI, drawing from funding by its member States. Finally, in applying any authorized measures, the GIJI would be subject to procedures of global administrative law, including oversight by an independent Appellate Tribunal.

Many of these procedures would not need to be invoked. We expect that the mere threat of compulsory licensing would accomplish a great deal, without its frequent exercise. Much good would therefore be done, at low cost and without incursions on state sovereignty or frequent use of coercion.

Implications for methodology

This chapter is, to my knowledge, unique in the literature on enhancement. It focuses squarely on the institutional causes of a central problem in the ethics of enhancement—the problem of justice in diffusion—shows that this is only one instance of a more general problem of justice in the diffusion of beneficial innovations, and then develops a detailed institutional proposal for how to cope with that problem. The institutional proposal is grounded in a philosophical analysis of the problem of justice in diffusion, but also relies on the expertise in institutional design of a political scientist who specializes in international institutions and the valuable contributions of an international lawyer.

Several years ago, I came to the conclusion that the present volume would have to include a chapter that offered concrete policy recommendations for coping with issues of distributive justice. I was also convinced that it was important to avoid "enhancement exceptionalism" and instead to view the problems that enhancements raise in the broader context of justice in innovation as one important aspect of the ethics of development. As I struggled to write (and rewrite) that chapter I soon realized that my skills as philosopher were inadequate to the task. I was fortunate to enlist Robert O. Keohane to co-author a paper that could serve as a pilot for the chapter but which would be able to stand on its own. Eventually it became clear to us that a credible global institutional proposal of the sort we were devising needed to take into account the realities of existing international law. When Anthony Cole generously supplied us with comments on a version of the paper I presented at his university, Keohane and I eagerly invited him to join us in writing a new version of the paper that took the international legal landscape into account. The history of this chapter vividly demonstrates the need for interdisciplinary cooperation in developing concrete, realistic responses to the challenges of enhancement.

Some bioethicists will no doubt react with puzzlement (or even hostility) to the real-world orientation and attention to detail of this chapter's approach. Expressing discomfort is one thing, being able to articulate a superior alternative to the hard work of truly practical thinking is another. In my judgment, progress in the enhancement debate requires detailed institutional proposals for coping with the risks of enhancement, including possible negative impacts on justice, and this in turn requires an admission that the toolbox of philosopher bioethicists is not adequate to the task.

In Chapter One, I argued that it is time for the enhancement debate to get beyond the pros and cons stage and begin to explore concrete, practical solutions to the ethical problems that will arise with the widespread use of enhancements. In the present chapter I have tried to show what it means to take that suggestion seriously. In the middle chapters of this volume, I argued that productive thinking about enhancement must be grounded in evolutionary biology. I think it should now be clear that coming to grips with the ethics of biomedical enhancement will require a new way of thinking. Philosophers who wish to make a contribution to the next stage of the debate will have to adopt a different methodology. They will have to draw on the best work in the biological sciences; but they will also need to think institutionally and be willing to descend from the world of abstract argumentation to the real world of institutions, incentives, and power.

The right sort of philosophical thinking is a necessary component of a morally sensitive and realistic response to the promise and perils of biomedical enhancement, but it is far from sufficient. In the end, whether biomedical augmentations of various human *capacities* result in improvements in *human well-being* will depend on whether ordinary people, in their capacities as citizens participating in democratic political processes, are willing to avoid the temptation to find false comfort in stirring rhetoric and catchy slogans, and do the hard work of thinking clearly about enhancement. To cope with biomedical enhancements, we will need to enhance our skills of practical reasoning and our ability to translate the conclusions we arrive at into responsible personal behavior and effective collective action. In the short run, at least, we will have to do this without the aid of biomedical enhancements.

Notes

1. An important, though as I shall argue, partial exception is the work of Thomas Pogge in his Patent 2 proposal, which is discussed in the paper on which this chapter draws. See note 2.
2. My characterization of the GIJI proposal in this chapter is a truncated version of that set out in Allen Buchanan, Tony Cole, and Robert O. Keohane (forthcoming), "Justice in the Diffusion of Innovation," Journal of Political Philosophy, which includes a comparison of the GIJI with Thomas Pogge's proposal for a "Patent 2," as a response to the essential medicines problem.
3. See, for example, Francis Fukuyama (2002), *Our Posthuman Future* (New York: Farrar, Straus and Giroux), pp. 9–10.
4. Anders Sandberg, Nick Bostrom (2006), "Converging Cognitive Enhancements," *Annals of the New York Academy of Sciences* 1093: 201–227; Nick Bostrom (2008), "Smart Policy: Cognitive Enhancement in the Public Interest," in *Reshaping the Human Condition: Exploring Human Enhancement*, Leo Zonneveld, Huub Dijstelblowem, and Danielle Ringoir (eds.) (The Hague, Netherlands and London: Rathenau Institute, British Embassy Science & Innovation Network, and Parliamentary Office of Science and Technology), pp. 29–36.
5. Allen Buchanan (1984), "The Right to a Decent Minimum of Health Care," *Philosophy & Public Affairs* 13(1): 55–78; Normal Daniels (2001), "Justice, Health, and Healthcare," *The American Journal of Bioethics* 1(2): 2–16; Dan Brock (2003), "Ethical Issues in the Use of Cost-Effectiveness Analysis for the Prioritization of Health Care Resources," in *Making Choices in Health:*

WHO Guide to Cost-Effectiveness Analysis, T. Edejer, *et al.* (eds.) (Geneva: World Health Organization), pp. 289–312.

6. Gopal Sreenivasan (2002), "International Justice and Health: A Proposal," *Ethics and International Affairs* 16: 81–90.

7. Michael Walzer (1983), *Spheres of Justice: A Defense of Pluralism and Equality* (Basic Books), Chapter 1.

8. According to some democratic theorists, what might be called basic political equality—having secure standing as an equal participant in the most fundamental political processes in one's society—is itself a requirement of justice, because it is required for a proper public recognition of the equality of citizens. On this view, inequalities in political power that are incompatible with or that tend to undermine this fundamental equality are unjust, independently of their tendency to produce other bad effects, including extreme deprivations, violations of particular civil and political rights, or distributive unfairness.
    See Thomas Christiano (2008), *The Constitution of Equality: Democratic Authority and Its Limits* (Oxford: Oxford University Press).

9. By free-rider problems I mean situations where the collective action needed to produce some benefit fails to occur because individuals refrain from contributing because they think that they will be able to enjoy the benefit if they don't contribute. By assurance problems I mean situations where the collective action needed to produce some benefit fails to occur, not because individuals attempt to free-ride, but because they lack assurance that (enough) others will contribute.

10. It should be noted that when "monopoly pricing" is referred to in the current article, this includes the partial or complete refusal to sell in a given market by an IPR holder, as this refusal is based upon an inability to receive the monopoly prices insisted upon.

11. On institutions see Stephen D. Krasner (ed.) (1983), *International Regimes* (Cambridge, MA: MIT Press), introduction; Robert O. Keohane (1989), *International Institutions and State Power* (Boulder, CO: Westview). On accountability see Ruth Grant and Robert O. Keohane (2005), "Accountability and abuses of power in world politics," *American Political Science Review,* 99(1): 29–43.

12. Geoffrey Brennan and Philip Pettit (2004), *The Economy of Esteem* (New York: Cambridge University Press).

13. The combination of notice and comment procedures with judicial review of due process is a feature of administrative law, as developed in the United States since the Administrative Procedures Act of 1946, and now spreading to international organizations. See Benedict Kingsbury, Nico Krisch, and Richard Stewart (2005), "The Emergence of Global Administrative Law," *Law and Contemporary Problems* 68(3/4): 15–62.

14. Article 5 of the Articles of Agreement of the International Bank for Reconstruction and Development, the largest unit in the World Bank

Group, provides that 20 percent of the subscription of each member is subject to call when needed for ordinary obligations of the Bank, and 80 percent is basically held in reserve to guarantee loans issued by the Bank. For the Articles of Agreement, see the World Bank website.

15. Where this includes the possibility of extra payment necessary to secure the cooperation of IPR holders in cases in which the IPR holder possessed non-public information essential for the manufacture of the licensed product.

16. Hedley Bull (1977), *The Anarchical Society* (New York: Columbia University Press), p. 8.

17. Naturally, the language used to describe the declaration is only intended to convey the substance of the declaration, and the precise wording of the document itself would need to be different.

ACKNOWLEDGEMENTS

This book is an expansion of the 2009 Oxford Uehiro Lectures, which I delivered in Oxford in 2009. I am deeply grateful to the Uehiro Foundation for Ethics and Education for this honor. By funding the Lectures and the Uehiro Centres for Practical Ethics in Tokyo and in Oxford, the Uehiro Foundation has been a major force in the development of contemporary Practical Ethics. The reach of the Uehiro Foundation's activities is global. Thanks to the leadership of its Chairman, Mr. Eiji Uehiro, there has been a special emphasis on the cross-cultural study of ethical issues.

I have benefited greatly from attending several international conferences sponsored by the Uehiro Foundation. A hallmark of Foundation activities is the creation of an atmosphere in which scholars from different religious and philosophical traditions can come together to engage in ethical inquiry that is rigorous and critical, but also always mutually respectful.

During the four months leading up to my Uehiro Lectures, I was fortunate to be a Leverhulme Visiting Professor at Oxford. I am grateful to the Leverhulme Foundation, to Julian Savulescu, Director of the Oxford Uehiro Centre, for nominating me for this honor, and to Andrew Goudie, Master of St Cross, for making my stay at his college so rewarding and enjoyable. St Cross provided delightful accommodation, excellent logistical support, and a stimulating intellectual environment.

As I hope the endnotes in the text of this book will indicate, I have profited from the work of many people in working out my ideas on enhancement. I am particularly indebted to the following members of the Oxford Uehiro Centre, with whom I had many fruitful conversations about enhancement during my stay in Oxford: Nick Bostrom, Steve Clarke, Roger Crisp, Alexandre Erler, Barbro Froding, Tom Douglas, Kei Hiruta, Ingmar Persson, Janet Radcliffe-Richards, Julian Savulescu, and Mark Sheehan. I learned a great deal from all of them. One aspect of Julian Savulescu's outstanding leadership as Director of the Centre is that he has helped to create an environment in which there is an optimal mix of independent thought and cooperation.

A number of people were kind enough to give me comments on the thinking that culminated in this book. I owe a special debt of gratitude to Nicholas Agar, David Crawford, Tom Douglas, and Russell Powell for their valuable comments on drafts of chapters. Russell Powell played an especially influential role in shaping my thinking by helping me to realize how vital evolutionary biology is to the topic of biomedical enhancement.

Peter Momtchiloff, the editor for Oxford's Uehiro Lectures volumes, provided valuable guidance as I worked through the process of deciding what sort of volume this should be. He was also accessible and supportive.

Thanks are also due for permissions to draw on several published articles: to The Johns Hopkins University Press for "Enhancement and the Ethics of Human Development," which appeared in *The Kennedy Institute of Ethics Journal*, 18, no. 1, 2008, pp. 1–34; to Blackwell Publishing for "Human Nature and Enhancement," which appeared in *Bioethics*, vol. 23, no. 3, 2009, pp.141–150; to Blackwell Publishing for "Moral Status and Human Enhancement," which appeared in *Philosophy & Public Affairs*, vol. 37, no. 4, 2009, pp. 346–381; and to Blackwell Publishing for "Justice in the Diffusion of Innovations" (co-authored with Robert O. Keohane and Anthony Cole), which appeared in *The Journal of Political Philosophy*, vol. 19, 2011.

INDEX